# The DIABETES seafood cookbook

## Fresh, Healthy, Low-Fat Cooking

# BARBARA SEELIG-BROWN

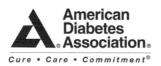

American Diabetes Association.
Cure • Care • Commitment®

Director, Book Publishing, Robert Anthony; Managing Editor, Book Publishing, Abe Ogden; Editor, Rebekah Renshaw; Production Manager, Melissa Sprott; Composition, ADA; Cover Design, Pixiedesign, Inc.; Printer, Transcontinental Printing

Printed in Canada
1 3 5 7 9 10 8 6 4 2

The suggestions and information contained in this publication are generally consistent with the Clinical Practice Recommendations and other policies of the American Diabetes Association, but they do not represent the policy or position of the Association or any of its boards or committees. Reasonable steps have been taken to ensure the accuracy of the information presented. However, the American Diabetes Association cannot ensure the safety or efficacy of any product or service described in this publication. Individuals are advised to consult a physician or other appropriate health care professional before undertaking any diet or exercise program or taking any medication referred to in this publication. Professionals must use and apply their own professional judgment, experience, and training and should not rely solely on the information contained in this publication before prescribing any diet, exercise, or medication. The American Diabetes Association—its officers, directors, employees, volunteers, and members—assumes no responsibility or liability for personal or other injury, loss, or damage that may result from the suggestions or information in this publication.

∞ The paper in this publication meets the requirements of the ANSI Standard Z39.48-1992 (permanence of paper).

ADA titles may be purchased for business or promotional use or for special sales. To purchase more than 50 copies of this book at a discount, or for custom editions of this book with your logo, contact the American Diabetes Association at the address below, at booksales@diabetes.org, or by calling 703-299-2046.

American Diabetes Association
1701 North Beauregard Street
Alexandria, Virginia 22311

**Library of Congress Cataloging-in-Publication Data**

Selig-Brown, Barbara.
The diabetes seafood cookbook / Barbara Selig-Brown.
    p. cm.
Includes bibliographical references and index.
ISBN 978-1-58040-302-3 (alk. paper)
1. Diabetes--Diet therapy--Recipes. 2. Cookery (Seafood) I. American Diabetes Association. II. Title.

RC662.S45 2009
641.5'6314--dc22
                        2008055030

# TABLE OF CONTENTS

# Dedication

*For my mom, with heartfelt thanks for the memorable meals that inspired my love of cooking for family and friends. I wish we could cook together again.*

# Acknowledgments

There are so many wonderful folks to acknowledge in making this book happen.

I'd like to thank my husband, Alan Brown, and our family for their patience and tasting expertise, especially those nights when you thought you were going to grow fins if you ate more fish.

Rebekah Renshaw, my editor, for being so pleasant and professional to work with; Rob Anthony for being receptive; and the other ADA staff members, Abe Ogden, Melissa Sprott, and Heschel Falek for making this book a reality. I'd also like to thank the food photographer Taran Z, and the food stylist, Lisa Cherkasky, who created the lovely photographs of the recipes in this book.

Kathy O'Shea and Jen Olsen for their assistance in the kitchen and the office.

Daniella Massey of The Spice Hunter and Anne North of Phillips Seafood for their support.

All those who offered their suggestions during the initial book proposal phase: Ouida Brown; Marion Brown; Marilyn Witte Goldbard; Sue Sell of Cook 'N' Tell; Tim Cebula of *Cooking Light*; Mary Finckenor, MA, RD, CDE; Kathy Tigue, RD, CDE; Diana Lawrence of Romo Books; and Sarah Baurle.

# INTRODUCTION

# Fish Know-How

Let's get cooking!

We all know that we should incorporate more fish into our diet. It is low in fat, high in protein, and contains valuable vitamins and minerals, as well as omega-3 oils, which are polyunsaturated. The type of fat we consume is relevant for a heart-healthy diet, that being less than 30% of all calories from fat with less than 10% coming from saturated fats. Studies have been done showing that a healthy diet featuring a variety of foods, including fish, can actually decrease the risk for coronary disease and certain cancers, as well as increase longevity. Since people with diabetes are also at risk for heart disease, fish is an important component.

Many people shy away from cooking fish because they just don't know how to buy, store, or cook it. Let's start with some basics so that we can keep it simple. Dinner at home should be enjoyable, and some fish basics will make that possible. Keeping it simple and fresh will also help achieve that goal. One of the best things about fish is that you don't need to do a lot to it; in fact, you don't want to overpower it. Of course, if you don't like fish, then disguising it with strong flavors is for you. A variety of recipes will be presented in this book.

## SHOPPING AND STORAGE

Fish should smell sweet or smell like the ocean. Smelly fish is old and not for you. When you look at the fish counter, it should look appetizing and fresh. The fish you see should be shiny, firm, and if whole, the eyes should be clear. Many supermarkets do not even carry whole fish because the demand for them is not as great as more common varieties like shellfish and fillets. Whole fish is generally available at a good fish store and is worth the effort to find it. If you are courageous you can give the recipes in the Whole Fish chapter a try.

Just like meat, fish on the bone is more tender and succulent. When you are shopping, you should buy your fish last and ask for it to be put on ice so that you don't have to worry about food safety. When you arrive home, put it away first. You can store it either wrapped in waxed paper, in a tightly sealed plastic container, or on top of a bed of ice placed in a colander in a bowl. Use fresh fish within a day of purchasing. Always check with the fish manager as to when the fish was delivered to the store. A good fish manager will tell you when it comes in and will also tell you what the best value is on the day you are shopping. I always give the experts their due and rely on them to help me get just what I need.

## COOKING & TESTING FOR DONENESS

A general rule of thumb for cooking fish is 10 minutes per inch of thickness. A one-inch thick fillet should take at least 10 minutes to cook. Another way to check is to see if it flakes when pierced with a fork; however, for some varieties, such as salmon and tuna, this would be considered overcooked. A meat thermometer is your best friend. To retain flavor, tuna and swordfish should be cooked to an internal temperature of 125°. Fish steaks, fillets, or whole fish should be cooked to an internal temperature of 140°. White flesh fish should look opaque when cooked. Clams, mussels, and oysters are cooked until their shells open. Discard any that do not open. Shellfish like shrimp and lobster are cooked until pink and opaque.

## THE RECIPES

The recipes in this book were developed with the thought that you could interchange the cooking methods, sauces, marinades, and side dishes. Some will be one-dish meals, while others will have serving suggestions. The chapter on Rounding Out the Meal is helpful in deciding what to serve to complete your menu. There is even a dessert!

## TYPES OF FISH

There are endless varieties of fish to choose from. Depending on what part of the country you live in and also what season we are in, certain species will or will not be available. You can purchase some of the harder-to-find varieties of fish and seafood directly from the fishermen through the Internet.

The most commonly eaten fish are salmon and tuna. There are many recipes using these varieties. You should decide what your feelings are on wild vs. farm raised, along with the varieties that are surrounded by the mercury controversy, such as tuna and swordfish. Yes, wild salmon is more nutritious than farm-raised, but if it is not available or the cost is prohibitive, then farm-raised will do. There are also social responsibilities to consider. Do you feel right knowing that a specific variety like Chilean sea bass might become extinct because it is overfished? I choose not to overeat this variety, but I know many people that feel that if it is in the stores, you should buy it.

Remember one thing, research is constantly changing and nutrition is constantly being re-evaluated.

Methyl mercury is a naturally occurring substance in our environment; the main sources are from power plants that burn fossil fuels and coal. Mercury accumulates in streams, oceans, rivers, and lakes. After a chemical transformation, it becomes toxic. Fish absorb the mercury by feeding on aquatic organisms. Mercury is more prominent in larger fish, as they survive by eating the smaller ones. Older fish also contain more mercury than younger ones, because they are exposed longer. Of course, we can't really tell how old a fish is, so we need to exercise our own good judgment.

Vulnerable and sensitive populations, such as young children, pregnant women, women of childbearing age who might become pregnant, or nursing mothers should avoid excessive consumption of high-mercury fish. The most widely accepted recommendation for women of childbearing age is 8 oz of uncooked fish or 6 oz of cooked fish per week and 3 oz of uncooked and 2 oz of cooked fish for children. There are differing opinions on just how much fish containing higher levels of mercury should be consumed by anyone. For more information, consult FDA data, Mercury Levels in Seafood Species, or the EPA, which is endorsed by the National Academy of Sciences.

# MERCURY CONTENT IN FISH

## Fish High in Mercury

King Mackerel

Shark

Swordfish

Tile fish

Tuna

## Fish Low in Mercury

| | | |
|---|---|---|
| Catfish | Lobster | Scallops |
| Cod | Mahi Mahi | Shrimp |
| Crab | Ocean Perch | Spiny Lobster |
| Flounder/Sole | Oysters | Tilapia |
| Haddock | Rainbow Trout | Farmed Trout |
| Herring | Sardines | Farmed Salmon |

# Chapter 1:

# STARTERS

*Hot dips and spreads are always a big hit because they are so easy to make.*

*This **Crab and Artichoke Dip** is a recipe you can enjoy without any guilt.*

## Serves 48 / Serving Size: 1 tsp
# crab and artichoke dip

Cooking spray

**8 oz** crabmeat (can, pouch, or frozen)

**10 oz** frozen artichoke hearts, chopped

**3 Tbsp** Parmigiano-Reggiano

**2 Tbsp** light mayonnaise

**1/4 cup** plain nonfat yogurt

**1** lemon, juiced

**1/4 tsp** salt

**1/4 tsp** freshly ground black pepper

1. Preheat oven to 400°.

2. Spray baking dish with nonstick cooking spray. In large bowl, combine all ingredients. Pour into baking dish. Bake 30 minutes.

3. Serve with low-fat plain crackers, such as water crackers or whole-grain Melba toast.

## Cook's Tip

*Frozen artichoke hearts work better than canned because they are the closest to fresh, and don't contain any preservatives.*

EXCHANGES/CHOICES: 1 FREE FOOD
CALORIES 10, CALORIES FROM FAT 0,
TOTAL FAT 0 G, SATURATED FAT 0.1 G, TRANS FAT 0 G,
CHOLESTEROL 5 MG, SODIUM 25 MG, TOTAL CARBOHYDRATE 1 G,
DIETARY FIBER 0 G, SUGARS 0 G, PROTEIN 1 G

*This delicious Garlic Shrimp on a Cucumber Flower appetizer is beautiful to look at as well as figure friendly. Your guests will love it.*

**Serves 8 / Serving Size: 3 pieces**

# garlic shrimp on a cucumber flower

**1 lb** medium shrimp, peeled and deveined

**1** lemon, juiced

**2 cloves** garlic, crushed and minced to a paste

**2 Tbsp** extra virgin olive oil

**1/2 cup** chopped dill (additional for garnish)

**1/4 tsp** fine sea salt

**1/8 tsp** freshly ground pepper

**1** large English cucumber (enough to make 24 slices)

1. Steam shrimp in large pot with steamer basket insert. Cook just until pink, about 5–6 minutes.

2. Mix in lemon juice, garlic, olive oil, chopped dill, salt, and pepper. Marinate shrimp in this mixture for at least 1 hour and up to 24 hours. Refrigerate while marinating.

3. Scrub cucumber well. Take a fork and run it up and down the outside of cucumber to make a decorative edge. Slice cucumber into 24 rounds.

4. Place one piece of shrimp on a cucumber slice and garnish with another sprig of fresh dill. Cover and refrigerate until serving time.

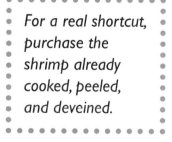

## Cook's Tip

*For a real shortcut, purchase the shrimp already cooked, peeled, and deveined.*

EXCHANGES/CHOICES: 1 LEAN MEAT, 1/2 FAT
CALORIES 65, CALORIES FROM FAT 25,
TOTAL FAT 3 G, SATURATED FAT 0.5 G, TRANS FAT 0 G,
CHOLESTEROL 65 MG, SODIUM 135 MG, TOTAL CARBOHYDRATE 2 G,
DIETARY FIBER 0 G, SUGARS 1 G, PROTEIN 7 G

*These **Lobster & Mango Salad Tarts** have a surprise sweetness and are loaded with Vitamin C for added health benefits.*

**Serves 4 / Serving Size: 1/4 recipe**

# lobster & mango salad tarts

**8 oz** plain low-fat yogurt

**1 lb** lobster meat, steamed, cooled, and diced

**1/4 cup** finely minced shallot

**1** large mango, diced into 1/4-inch pieces

**1 cup** roughly chopped cilantro

**1** lemon, juiced

**1 package** mini phyllo tart shells (can be purchased in most grocery stores)

1. Drain yogurt through a cheesecloth or coffee filter placed in a strainer that has been placed in a bowl. This will reduce whey and make a thicker consistency.

2. Mix lobster, shallot, mango, cilantro, lemon, and half the yogurt. Blend well. Add remaining yogurt as necessary for desired consistency.

3. Serve in a mini phyllo tart shell or over mixed greens.

## Cook's Tip

*Mango are ripe when they are soft to the touch. If they have been handled a lot in the store, they do not always ripen well at home, so purchase them when you are ready to use them.*

**EXCHANGES/CHOICES: 2 STARCH, 1 FRUIT, 3 LEAN MEAT, 2 FAT**
**CALORIES 445, CALORIES FROM FAT 145,**
**TOTAL FAT 16 G, SATURATED FAT 0.7 G, TRANS FAT 0 G,**
**CHOLESTEROL 85 MG, SODIUM 650 MG, TOTAL CARBOHYDRATE 48 G,**
**DIETARY FIBER 2 G, SUGARS 15 G, PROTEIN 27 G**

*Mediterranean Grilled Sardines* make for a great appetizer at an outdoor party. Your guests can mingle while you prepare this dish.

**Serves 4 / Serving Size: I sardine**

# mediterranean grilled sardines

**1 Tbsp** extra virgin olive oil

**1/4 tsp** fine sea salt

**1/4 tsp** freshly ground black pepper

**1 Tbsp** fresh marjoram leaves

**1 Tbsp** fresh rosemary leaves

**1 Tbsp** fresh lemon zest

**4** fresh sardines

1. Mix olive oil, salt, pepper, marjoram, rosemary, and lemon zest together. Toss sardines with this mixture. Refrigerate for several hours to allow flavors to blend.

2. Preheat grill to high. Reduce heat to medium and grill sardines 3–4 minutes on each side.

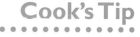

## Cook's Tip

*These fish are more popular in Mediterranean cooking so you might have to go to a specialty or seafood store to find them.*

EXCHANGES/CHOICES: 2 LEAN MEAT, 1 1/2 FAT
CALORIES 160, CALORIES FROM FAT 100,
TOTAL FAT 11 G, SATURATED FAT 2.1 G, TRANS FAT 0 G,
CHOLESTEROL 45 MG, SODIUM 220 MG, TOTAL CARBOHYDRATE 1 G,
DIETARY FIBER 0 G, SUGARS 0 G, PROTEIN 14 G

*Crab Cakes vary from chef to chef, but I like these* **Mini Crab Cakes with Horseradish**, *because the sweetness of the crab really comes through.*

## Serves 9 / Serving size: 2 crab cakes
# mini crab cakes with horseradish

**8 oz** pasteurized crabmeat (backfin is best)
**1/2 cup** Italian-style bread crumbs
**1/4 cup** roughly chopped scallions
**1 Tbsp** fresh lemon juice
**1/2 tsp** hot sauce
**1/4 tsp** fine sea salt
**2** egg whites
**1/4 tsp** fresh black pepper
**1 cup** corn flakes

**horseradish sauce**
**1/2 cup** plain low-fat yogurt
**1 tsp** prepared horseradish

1. Preheat oven to 450°.

2. Mix together crabmeat, bread crumbs, scallions, lemon juice, hot sauce, sea salt, egg whites, and black pepper. Mixture should be dry enough to form balls. If not, add more bread crumbs.

3. Finely crush corn flakes in food processor. Roll crab mixture into small balls and then into corn flakes. Bake on parchment-lined baking sheet until golden, approximately 10 minutes.

4. Drain yogurt through cheesecloth or coffee filter set in a colander for 20 minutes. Mix with horseradish and serve over crab cakes.

EXCHANGES/CHOICES: 1/2 STARCH, 1/2 LEAN MEAT
CALORIES 70, CALORIES FROM FAT 10,
TOTAL FAT 1 G, SATURATED FAT 0.3 G, TRANS FAT 0 G,
CHOLESTEROL 35 MG, SODIUM 310 MG, TOTAL CARBOHYDRATE 8 G,
DIETARY FIBER 0 G, SUGARS 2 G, PROTEIN 7 G

*These **Salmon & Chive Pinwheels** not only look great and will impress your guests, but they're tasty little appetizers as well.*

**Serves 24 / Serving Size: 1 pinwheel**

# salmon & chive pinwheels

**8 oz** smoked salmon, thinly sliced

**4 oz** light cream cheese

**2 Tbsp** chives, snipped or chopped (additional for garnish)

**1 loaf** cocktail bread (pumpernickel or rye)

1. Lay salmon out on counter so that you have 2 squares, about 4 oz each.

2. Mix cream cheese and chives together and spread 1/2 of this mixture on each square of salmon.

3. Roll like a jellyroll and freeze for 30 minutes. (This will make slicing easier.)

4. Mark 24 slices before beginning. Slice with a serrated knife and place on a piece of cocktail bread. Garnish with chopped fresh chives.

5. Serve immediately or cover tightly and serve within a few hours.

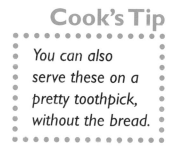

## Cook's Tip

*You can also serve these on a pretty toothpick, without the bread.*

EXCHANGES/CHOICES: 1 LEAN MEAT
CALORIES 40, CALORIES FROM FAT 15,
TOTAL FAT 1.5 G, SATURATED FAT 0.8 G, TRANS FAT 0 G,
CHOLESTEROL 5 MG, SODIUM 140 MG, TOTAL CARBOHYDRATE 3 G,
DIETARY FIBER 0 G, SUGARS 0 G, PROTEIN 3 G

*These tropically inspired **Salmon Kebabs with Pineapple & Mint** will instantly transport you back to summertime.*

**Serves 12 / Serving Size: 1 kebab**

# salmon kebabs
## with pineapple & mint

**12** wooden skewers (6 to 10 inches long)

**1 Tbsp** clover or orange blossom honey

**2** lemons, juiced

**1 Tbsp** extra virgin olive oil

**1/4 tsp** fine sea salt

**1/4 tsp** freshly ground black pepper

**2 Tbsp** chopped fresh mint

**1 lb** salmon fillet, skin removed, cut into 1-inch cubes

**1** pineapple, cut into 1-inch cubes

1. Place skewers in a shallow bowl of water and soak to prevent charring during grilling.

2. Mix honey, lemon juice, olive oil, salt, pepper, and mint together for marinade. Place salmon and pineapple in marinade for at least 20 minutes and up to 2 hours.

3. Thread salmon and pineapple equally on each of 12 skewers, starting with salmon and ending with pineapple.

4. Preheat grill pan. Place kebabs on pan and cook 5 minutes, turning as salmon begins to brown.

EXCHANGES/CHOICES: 1/2 FRUIT, 1 LEAN MEAT, 1/2 FAT
CALORIES 100, CALORIES FROM FAT 40,
TOTAL FAT 4.5 G, SATURATED FAT 0.7 G, TRANS FAT 0 G,
CHOLESTEROL 25 MG, SODIUM 70 MG, TOTAL CARBOHYDRATE 7 G,
DIETARY FIBER 1 G, SUGARS 5 G, PROTEIN 8 G

*Frozen clams are a dependable freezer item and can help you put this **Sautéed Escarole with Clams** together in no time.*

**Serves 4 / Serving Size: 1/4 recipe**

# sautéed escarole with clams

**1 Tbsp** extra virgin olive oil
**1 small head** escarole, washed and chopped
**2 large cloves** garlic, crushed and peeled
**1 (16 oz) bag** frozen clams on the half shell (about 24 clams)
**1/4 tsp** crushed red pepper flakes, to taste (optional)

1. Thinly film sauté pan with extra virgin olive oil.

2. Add escarole and garlic. Cook until escarole is wilted and tender. Add clams, cover, and cook until clams are heated thoroughly, about 3 minutes.

3. Place escarole and clams on a plate and sprinkle the optional crushed red pepper flakes on top. Serve with whole-grain crusty bread.

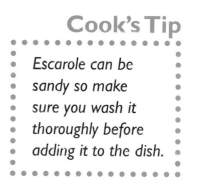

## Cook's Tip

*Escarole can be sandy so make sure you wash it thoroughly before adding it to the dish.*

EXCHANGES/CHOICES: 1 CARBOHYDRATE, 5 LEAN MEAT
CALORIES 305, CALORIES FROM FAT 90,
TOTAL FAT 10 G, SATURATED FAT 1.2 G, TRANS FAT 0 G,
CHOLESTEROL 100 MG, SODIUM 190 MG, TOTAL CARBOHYDRATE 12 G,
DIETARY FIBER 3 G, SUGARS 8 G, PROTEIN 40 G

*A simple hors d'oeuvre, this Scallop Seviche Martini looks very elegant when served in a martini glass.*

**Serves 8 / Serving Size: 1/8 recipe**

# scallop seviche martini

**12 oz** bay scallops
**1 cup** freshly squeezed lime juice
**1/2 cup** finely chopped red onion
**1 small** ripe tomato, peeled and chopped
**1** fresh jalapeño pepper, seeded and finely
     minced (wear gloves)
**2 Tbsp** canola oil
**1 tsp** granulated sugar
**2 Tbsp** white wine vinegar
**1/2 cup** fresh cilantro leaves, coarsely chopped
**1/4 tsp** fine sea salt
**1/8 tsp** freshly ground white pepper

1. Place scallops in a dish and add just enough lime juice to cover. Refrigerate at least 5 hours (not more than 24). Stir several times while in refrigerator.

2. Add onion, tomato, jalapeño, oil, sugar, vinegar, cilantro, salt, and pepper to scallops. Toss gently. Cover and refrigerate until it's time to assemble.

3. Drain the scallops and spoon into the martini glass. Garnish with fresh cilantro (if desired).

## Cook's Tip

*For large parties, try using disposable martini glasses. It's cheaper than buying a bunch, and much easier to clean up afterwards.*

EXCHANGES/CHOICES: 1 LEAN MEAT, 1/2 FAT
CALORIES 80, CALORIES FROM FAT 35,
TOTAL FAT 4 G, SATURATED FAT 0.3 G, TRANS FAT 0 G,
CHOLESTEROL 15 MG, SODIUM 145 MG, TOTAL CARBOHYDRATE 4 G,
DIETARY FIBER 0 G, SUGARS 2 G, PROTEIN 7 G

*When I take **Shrimp and Goat Cheese Mousse** to parties, I always hear people say, "Wow! I wonder who made that?"*

**Serves 36 / Serving Size: 1 stuffed spear**

# shrimp and goat cheese mousse

**6 oz** goat cheese

**3 oz** light cream cheese

**2 Tbsp** fresh dill, chopped (additional for garnish)

**1 Tbsp** freshly grated orange zest

**3–4 heads** Belgium endive, washed and dried, leaves separated and kept whole

**36** medium shrimp, steamed, peeled, and deveined

1. Mix together goat cheese, cream cheese, dill, and orange zest.

2. Place 1 tsp of goat cheese mousse on the wider end of the endive. Top with a shrimp and a fresh sprig of dill.

3. Refrigerate until serving time.

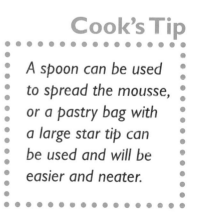

## Cook's Tip

*A spoon can be used to spread the mousse, or a pastry bag with a large star tip can be used and will be easier and neater.*

EXCHANGES/CHOICES: 1/2 FAT

CALORIES 25, CALORIES FROM FAT 15,

TOTAL FAT 1.5 G, SATURATED FAT 1.0 G, TRANS FAT 0 G,

CHOLESTEROL 15 MG, SODIUM 40 MG, TOTAL CARBOHYDRATE 0 G,

DIETARY FIBER 0 G, SUGARS 0 G, PROTEIN 2 G

*Spiedini is the Italian word for kebab. You can use small skewers for appetizers or large skewers for entrées for this* **Shrimp & Scallop Spiedini**.

**Serves 8 / Serving Size: 1/8 recipe**

# shrimp & scallop spiedini

**1 package** wooden skewers, 6–12 inches
**1** lemon, juiced
**1 Tbsp** chopped fresh rosemary
**1 clove** garlic, finely minced
**1 tsp** extra virgin olive oil
**1/4 tsp** fine sea salt
**1/4 tsp** freshly ground black pepper
**1/2 lb** large shrimp
**1/2 lb** large scallops

1. Place skewers in a shallow bowl of water and soak to prevent charring during grilling.

2. Mix together lemon juice, rosemary, garlic, olive oil, salt, and pepper. Place the seafood in the marinade for 20 minutes to 2 hours. Refrigerate while marinating. Thread shrimp and scallops on skewers.

3. Preheat grill, grill pan, or broiler. Cook 3–5 minutes until shrimp are pink and scallops begin to brown.

## Cook's Tip

*Don't overmarinate the seafood or you will have something similar to seviche, which is seafood cooked from the acid in the dish.*

EXCHANGES/CHOICES: 1 LEAN MEAT
CALORIES 65, CALORIES FROM FAT 15,
TOTAL FAT 1.5 G, SATURATED FAT 0.3 G, TRANS FAT 0 G,
CHOLESTEROL 55 MG, SODIUM 180 MG, TOTAL CARBOHYDRATE 0 G,
DIETARY FIBER 0 G, SUGARS 0 G, PROTEIN 11 G

*The delicious filling for these* **Shrimp Scampi Mini Phyllo Tarts** *is at its best when made several hours prior to serving.*

**Serves 5 / Serving Size: 3 tarts**

# shrimp scampi mini phyllo tarts

**1 large clove** garlic
**1/8 tsp** salt
**1** lemon, juiced
**1 Tbsp** light mayonnaise
**1/2 cup** flat Italian parsley
**4 oz** cooked salad shrimp
**1 (2.1 oz) package** mini phyllo tart shells

1. Place one clove garlic on cutting board. Place the flat side of a chef's knife on top of the garlic. With your other hand, give the chef's knife a good strong whack over the garlic. Lift up the knife and remove the papery garlic skin. Sprinkle garlic with salt. Using the flat side of the chef's knife, rub the salt into the garlic, creating a creamy paste.

2. In a bowl, combine garlic paste with lemon juice, mayonnaise, and a pinch of salt until well blended. Add 1/4 cup chopped parsley and the salad shrimp. Stir. Cover and chill in refrigerator until ready to use.

3. When ready to serve, place 1 Tbsp of filling in each mini tart shell. Garnish with remainder of chopped parsley and freshly ground pepper.

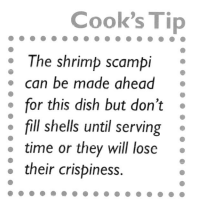

## Cook's Tip

*The shrimp scampi can be made ahead for this dish but don't fill shells until serving time or they will lose their crispiness.*

**EXCHANGES/CHOICES:** 1/2 STARCH, 1 LEAN MEAT
CALORIES 85, CALORIES FROM FAT 35,
TOTAL FAT 4 G, SATURATED FAT 0.2 G, TRANS FAT 0 G,
CHOLESTEROL 45 MG, SODIUM 175 MG, TOTAL CARBOHYDRATE 7 G,
DIETARY FIBER 0 G, SUGARS 0 G, PROTEIN 5 G

*Make this **Shrimp Stromboli** recipe ahead of time and keep it in your freezer and you'll have a quick party dish whenever you need one.*

**Serves 16 / Serving Size: 1 slice**

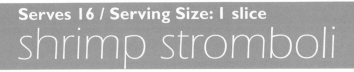

# shrimp stromboli

**1 package** prepared pizza dough

**1 (6 oz) bag** baby spinach

**1 (3 oz) package** sliced fresh mushrooms

**4 oz** frozen, peeled, deveined large shrimp, sliced in half horizontally

**1/4 cup** grated Grana Padano cheese

**1/2 cup** chopped chives

**1 tsp** extra virgin olive oil

1. Preheat oven to 375°.

2. Roll dough into rectangle. Layer spinach, mushrooms, shrimp, cheese, and chives on top of dough, leaving a 1-inch border on all sides. Begin rolling on one of the long sides. Roll tightly and make sure that you finish seam side down on a parchment-lined baking sheet. Brush with extra virgin olive oil for golden color.

3. Bake for 35–45 minutes or until golden. Cool at least 10 minutes before cutting.

## Cook's Tip

*Cooling this dish before cutting really makes a difference and gives you a "nicer slice."*

**EXCHANGES/CHOICES: 1 STARCH**
**CALORIES 90, CALORIES FROM FAT 15,**
**TOTAL FAT 1.5 G, SATURATED FAT 0.6 G, TRANS FAT 0 G,**
**CHOLESTEROL 10 MG, SODIUM 195 MG, TOTAL CARBOHYDRATE 15 G,**
**DIETARY FIBER 1 G, SUGARS 1 G, PROTEIN 5 G**

*Hearts of palm are full of Vitamin C. This* **Smoked Salmon & Hearts of Palm on Endive** *combines those benefits with the benefits of salmon.*

**Serves 24 / Serving Size: 1 piece**

# smoked salmon
## & hearts of palm on endive

**8 oz** fat-free cream cheese

**1/4 cup** fresh minced dill (additional sprigs for garnish)

**1** lemon, juiced

**3 heads** Belgian endive

**1 (10 oz)** can hearts of palm (about 6 pieces, approximately 4 inches in length)

**1 lb** smoked salmon, thinly sliced

**1/4 tsp** freshly ground pepper

1. Soften cream cheese at room temperature for about 20 minutes. Mix with minced dill and lemon juice.

2. Wash and dry the endive. Separate the leaves (spears). Cut hearts of palm into 1/4-inch-thick lengths. Wrap lengthwise in a piece of salmon.

3. Spread a thin layer of the cream cheese mixture on the endive leaf and top with the salmon-wrapped hearts of palm.

4. Garnish with a sprinkling of freshly ground black pepper and a piece of dill.

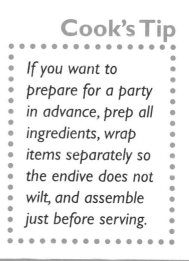

## Cook's Tip

*If you want to prepare for a party in advance, prep all ingredients, wrap items separately so the endive does not wilt, and assemble just before serving.*

EXCHANGES/CHOICES: 1 LEAN MEAT
CALORIES 40, CALORIES FROM FAT 10,
TOTAL FAT 1 G, SATURATED FAT 0.2 G, TRANS FAT 0 G,
CHOLESTEROL 5 MG, SODIUM 235 MG, TOTAL CARBOHYDRATE 2 G,
DIETARY FIBER 0 G, SUGARS 1 G, PROTEIN 5 G

*Spreads like this* **Smoked Salmon Spread** *are easy to make, and when you prepare them at home, they're tastier and healthier.*

**Serves 8 / Serving Size: 1/4 cup**

# smoked salmon spread

**1 cup** 1% cottage cheese
**1/2 cup** sliced hearts of palm
**1** lemon, juiced (divided use)
**2 Tbsp** minced shallot (about 1 small)
**4 oz** smoked salmon, roughly chopped
**1/4 cup** fresh dill

1. Place cottage cheese, hearts of palm, juice of 1/2 lemon, and shallot in food processor fitted with steel blade. Pulse until blended.

2. Add salmon and dill and pulse until salmon is evenly incorporated. Taste for seasoning and add remaining lemon if desired.

3. Serve with crackers or vegetables, such as sliced fennel, endive, or celery.

## Cook's Tip

*The sweet, mild flavor of the shallot is a nice change from the traditional onion. It compliments the salmon nicely in this dish.*

EXCHANGES/CHOICES: 1 LEAN MEAT
CALORIES 50, CALORIES FROM FAT 10,
TOTAL FAT 1 G, SATURATED FAT 0.3 G, TRANS FAT 0 G,
CHOLESTEROL 5 MG, SODIUM 250 MG, TOTAL CARBOHYDRATE 4 G,
DIETARY FIBER 0 G, SUGARS 3 G, PROTEIN 6 G

*These **Stuffed Clams** are the perfect finger food because the clam shell provides its own serving dish for fast, easy cleanup.*

**Serves 12 / Serving Size: 2 clams**

# stuffed clams

- **1 Tbsp** extra virgin olive oil
- **2 oz** pancetta, chopped
- **1** medium onion, minced
- **2 cloves** garlic, minced
- **2 cups** baby spinach, roughly chopped
- **1 cup** plain bread crumbs
- **1 cup** clam juice or vegetable stock
- **1 (16 oz) bag** frozen clams on the half shell (about 24 clams)
- **1/4 cup** finely grated Parmigiano-Reggiano

1. Place olive oil in a large nonstick skillet. Heat and add chopped pancetta, minced onion, and garlic. Cook until onion becomes translucent and pancetta is crispy.

2. Add baby spinach, bread crumbs, and clam juice. Mix well and cook approximately 3 minutes.

3. Top each clam with 1 tsp of this mixture and place on a baking sheet. Place in preheated oven and bake 15 minutes until golden brown.

4. Sprinkle with Parmigiano-Reggiano.

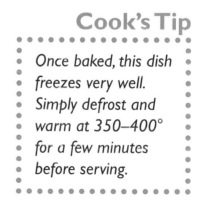

## Cook's Tip

*Once baked, this dish freezes very well. Simply defrost and warm at 350–400° for a few minutes before serving.*

EXCHANGES/CHOICES: 1/2 STARCH, 1 LEAN MEAT, 1/2 FAT
CALORIES 100, CALORIES FROM FAT 25,
TOTAL FAT 3 G, SATURATED FAT 0.7 G, TRANS FAT 0 G,
CHOLESTEROL 20 MG, SODIUM 200 MG, TOTAL CARBOHYDRATE 9 G,
DIETARY FIBER 1 G, SUGARS 2 G, PROTEIN 9 G

*This **Trout with Wild Mushrooms** recipe is an excellent first course that all of your guests are guaranteed to love.*

**Serves 4 / Serving Size: 1/4 recipe**

# trout with wild mushrooms

**1/4 cup** Wondra flour

**1/4 tsp** fine sea salt

**1/8 tsp** freshly ground black pepper

**1 lb** trout fillet

**1 Tbsp** extra virgin olive oil

**1 package** gourmet mushroom blend (about 3 oz)

**1/4 cup** dry white wine

1. Place Wondra in shallow dish or pie plate. Add salt and pepper. Dredge trout in flour.

2. Place olive oil in large nonstick sauté pan. Heat and melt butter. Add trout and cook first side until golden. Turn fish. While second side cooks, add mushrooms to pan surface. Sauté mushrooms and brown second side of fish.

3. Add 1/4 cup white wine, bring to boil, and then reduce heat to simmer. Cook 2–3 minutes to create sauce.

## Cook's Tip

*Using unsalted butter helps keep sodium down and also gives you more control of the sodium used in the dish.*

**EXCHANGES/CHOICES:** 1/2 CARBOHYDRATE, 3 LEAN MEAT, 1/2 FAT
**CALORIES** 205, **CALORIES FROM FAT** 70,
**TOTAL FAT** 8 G, **SATURATED FAT** 1.3 G, **TRANS FAT** 0 G,
**CHOLESTEROL** 65 MG, **SODIUM** 210 MG, **TOTAL CARBOHYDRATE** 7 G,
**DIETARY FIBER** 0 G, **SUGARS** 0 G, **PROTEIN** 25 G

*Truffles are one of life's many pleasures, so I am happy to include this delightful* **Truffled Scallops** *recipe in this book.*

**Serves 6 / Serving Size: 1/6 recipe**
# truffled scallops

**1 lb** bay scallops (frozen are acceptable)

**1 Tbsp** extra virgin olive oil

**1 clove** garlic

**2 Tbsp** minced shallots (about 1 large)

**5 oz** sliced cremini mushrooms

**1/4 cup** chicken stock

**1/4 cup** skim milk

**1/4 cup** whole-grain bread crumbs

**1/4 tsp** white truffle oil

**1/2 cup** minced fresh parsley

1. Defrost scallops in cold water for 20 minutes and pat dry.

2. Place extra virgin olive oil, garlic, shallots, and mushrooms in large sauté pan. Turn heat to high and sauté until mushrooms begin to soften and shallots are translucent.

3. Add scallops, chicken stock, milk, and bread crumbs. Mix well and cook 3 minutes until mixture is thickened. Stir in truffle oil and parsley.

4. Serve in 6 small ramekins.

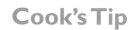

## Cook's Tip

*Truffle oil goes a long way. Purchase it in small bottles and keep it in a cool, dark place.*

EXCHANGES/CHOICES: 1/2 CARBOHYDRATE, 2 LEAN MEAT
CALORIES 115, CALORIES FROM FAT 30,
TOTAL FAT 3.5 G, SATURATED FAT 0.4 G, TRANS FAT 0 G,
CHOLESTEROL 30 MG, SODIUM 205 MG, TOTAL CARBOHYDRATE 5 G,
DIETARY FIBER 1 G, SUGARS 1 G, PROTEIN 15 G

# Chapter 2:

# SOUPS & SALADS

*I have always loved Asian Salads in restaurants, so I have figured out how to make it at home with this Asian Tuna Salad.*

**Serves 4 / Serving Size: 1/4 recipe**

# asian tuna salad

**16 oz** tuna steak
**1 tsp** canola oil
**1/4 cup** pignoli (pine nuts)
**1 medium head** napa cabbage,
    julienned (reserve a few large leaves)
**1** small heart of romaine (about 4 cups),
    julienned
**1/2 cup** snow peas, julienned

**salad dressing**
**2 tsp** dry mustard
**1/2 cup** rice wine vinegar
**1 tsp** peanut butter
**1 tsp** soy sauce
**1 Tbsp** sesame oil
**1 Tbsp** canola oil
**1/4 tsp** fine sea salt
**1/4** tsp freshly ground black pepper

1. Cut tuna into 1/2-inch-thick strips. Toss with canola oil. Sauté 3–4 minutes until golden. Set aside to cool.

2. Place pignoli in dry sauté pan. Heat to medium and cook until golden. Remove from pan to cool. Mix nuts with cabbage, heart of romaine, and snow peas.

3. Combine salad dressing ingredients. Toss with vegetable mixture. Add cooked tuna and toss gently.

4. Serve on leftover cabbage leaves.

EXCHANGES/CHOICES: 2 VEGETABLE, 4 LEAN MEAT, 4 FAT
CALORIES 400, CALORIES FROM FAT 235,
TOTAL FAT 26 G, SATURATED FAT 3.2 G, TRANS FAT 0 G,
CHOLESTEROL 40 MG, SODIUM 290 MG, TOTAL CARBOHYDRATE 12 G,
DIETARY FIBER 4 G, SUGARS 5 G, PROTEIN 32 G

*Make sure you have a good whole-grain bread to soak up all the*

*delicious broth in this* **Clams in Tomato Broth** *recipe.*

**Serves 2 / Serving Size: 1/2 recipe**

# clams in tomato broth

**1** fennel bulb, sliced thinly from tip to core

**4 large stems** fresh basil (with leaves)

**4 large stems** fresh oregano (with leaves)

**1** lemon, sliced into thin rounds

**4** plum tomatoes, roughly chopped

**1/8 tsp** sea salt

**1/8 tsp** black pepper

**2 dozen** cherrystone clams or 2 lb of mussels, scrubbed

**2 cups** dry white wine (Pinot Grigio or Sauvignon Blanc)

1. Layer fennel, herbs, lemon, tomatoes, salt, pepper, clams, and wine in a chef's pan (5–6 quart pan with tight-fitting lid). Cover. Bring to a boil and steam until clams open.

2. Serve in bowls with crusty Italian bread and broth.

## Cook's Tip

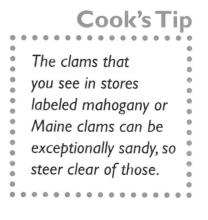

*The clams that you see in stores labeled mahogany or Maine clams can be exceptionally sandy, so steer clear of those.*

**EXCHANGES/CHOICES: 1/2 CARBOHYDRATE, 3 VEGETABLE, 5 LEAN MEAT**
**CALORIES 350, CALORIES FROM FAT 30,**
**TOTAL FAT 3.5 G, SATURATED FAT 0.3 G, TRANS FAT 0 G,**
**CHOLESTEROL 100 MG, SODIUM 390 MG, TOTAL CARBOHYDRATE 23 G,**
**DIETARY FIBER 5 G, SUGARS 14 G, PROTEIN 41 G**

*The convenience of pouch tuna makes this **Fillet of Tuna with White Soy Bean Salad** recipe a snap to prepare.*

**Serves 2 / Serving Size: 1/2 recipe**

# fillet of tuna
## with white soy bean salad

**1 Tbsp** extra virgin olive oil
**4 large cloves** garlic, sliced thinly lengthwise
**2** lemons (divided use)
**8 sprigs** fresh thyme
**1 cup** canned, drained, and rinsed white soy beans
**1/16 tsp** fine sea salt
**1/8 tsp** ground black pepper
**2 (4 oz)** tuna fillets, purchased in the pouch

1. Place olive oil in small sauté pan or saucepan. Add sliced garlic and turn to medium-high heat. Watch carefully and cook until golden. Remove garlic from oil with slotted spoon and place on paper towels. Set aside.

2. Mix the warm olive oil with juice from one lemon, thyme, and beans. Add salt and pepper. Set aside to allow flavors to blend. This salad can be made a day or two ahead of time.

3. Serve the white soy bean salad with 4 oz tuna fillet. Top with lemon slices.

### Cook's Tip

*If you cannot find white soy beans, you can use any white bean such as navy or cannellini.*

**EXCHANGES/CHOICES:** 1 STARCH, 4 LEAN MEAT, 1 1/2 FAT
**CALORIES** 325, **CALORIES FROM FAT** 145,
**TOTAL FAT** 16 G, **SATURATED FAT** 2.4 G, **TRANS FAT** 0 G,
**CHOLESTEROL** 40 MG, **SODIUM** 560 MG, **TOTAL CARBOHYDRATE** 12 G,
**DIETARY FIBER** 5 G, **SUGARS** 4 G, **PROTEIN** 37 G

*This beautiful **Grilled Escarole with Vinaigrette** salad can be made ahead of time and kept at room temperature until serving.*

**Serves 4 / Serving Size: 1/4 recipe**

# grilled escarole with vinaigrette

- **1 large head** escarole
- **4 Tbsp** extra virgin olive oil (divided use)
- **4 large cloves** garlic, sliced lengthwise
- **12** large shrimp (about 3/4 lb)
- **1 Tbsp** extra virgin olive oil
- **2** lemons (divided use)
- **2 tsp** fresh thyme leaves
- **1 cup** canned white beans, drained and rinsed well
- **1/4 tsp** fine sea salt
- **1/8 tsp** freshly ground pepper

1. Wash and dry escarole. Cut lengthwise into quarters, cutting through the core so that the leaves in each quarter remain intact. Set aside. Mix 2 Tbsp olive oil with garlic. Set aside.

2. Peel and devein shrimp. Spray with cooking spray. Spray escarole lightly with olive oil. Grill or sauté until lightly browned and only slightly wilted. Place on large platter or 4 dinner plates. Grill shrimp about 3 minutes on each side.

3. While shrimp is cooking, prepare bean mixture. Remove garlic from oil. Mix 1 Tbsp extra virgin olive oil, juice of one lemon, thyme, beans, salt, and pepper together.

4. Spoon 1/4 of bean mixture over each piece of escarole. Top with shrimp. Garnish with extra lemon slices, if desired.

## Cook's Tip

*Escarole can be very sandy, so it must be carefully washed. Fill your sink with water and swish the lettuce in the water to release dirt.*

**EXCHANGES/CHOICES: 1 STARCH, 2 LEAN MEAT, 1 FAT**
**CALORIES 205, CALORIES FROM FAT 70,**
**TOTAL FAT 8 G, SATURATED FAT 1.1 G, TRANS FAT 0 G,**
**CHOLESTEROL 90 MG, SODIUM 415 MG, TOTAL CARBOHYDRATE 17 G,**
**DIETARY FIBER 6 G, SUGARS 2 G, PROTEIN 17 G**

*Pomegranates are full of antioxidants, and the pomegranate syrup in this* **Grilled Tuna over Baby Greens** *adds a hint of tart-sweetness.*

**Serves 4 / Serving Size: 1/4 recipe**

# grilled tuna over baby greens

**pomegranate vinaigrette**
**1/4 cup** white balsamic vinegar
**2 tsp** pomegranate syrup
**1/4 tsp** fine sea salt
**1/8 tsp** freshly ground black pepper
**1/2 cup** extra virgin olive oil

**16 oz** tuna steak, cut into 4 portions
**8 cups** mixed greens (5 oz package)
**1 (11 oz) can** Mandarin orange slices,
      drained (about 3/4 cup)

1. Combine vinegar, pomegranate syrup, salt, and pepper in medium mixing bowl. Whisk. Slowly stream in the olive oil while you continue to whisk. Set aside.

2. Marinate tuna in 1 Tbsp pomegranate vinaigrette for about 20 minutes.

3. Heat grill pan. Drain tuna and place on grill pan. Grill first side about 4 minutes. Turn and grill second side to desired doneness.

4. Toss greens with 3 Tbsp pomegranate vinaigrette. Divide among 4 dinner plates. Top with grilled tuna and garnish with Mandarin orange slices.

### Cook's Tip

*Pomegranate syrup is available in specialty food stores or higher end grocery stores. If you can't find it, you can use pure cranberry juice instead.*

EXCHANGES/CHOICES: 1/2 Fat, 3 Lean Meat, 2 Fat
CALORIES 255, CALORIES FROM FAT 115,
TOTAL FAT 13 G, SATURATED FAT 2.4 G, TRANS FAT 0 G,
CHOLESTEROL 40 MG, SODIUM 95 MG, TOTAL CARBOHYDRATE 7 G,
DIETARY FIBER 1 G, SUGARS 6 G, PROTEIN 26 G

*Inspired by a soup in Bermuda that was so wonderful, I had to come home and try to recreate it in this **Italian Fish Soup**.*

**Serves 8 / Serving Size: 1/8 recipe**

# italian fish soup

- **2 tsp** extra virgin olive oil
- **1 cup** onion, chopped
- **1 cup** celery, chopped
- **1 cup** carrot, sliced
- **2 cups** Yukon Gold potatoes, peeled and diced
- **3 cloves** garlic, minced
- **1 cup** fresh basil, chopped
- **1/2 cup** fresh oregano, roughly chopped
- **1/4 tsp** fine sea salt
- **1/4 tsp** freshly ground pepper
- **1 (28 oz) can** diced tomatoes
- **1** green bell pepper, diced
- **1/4 cup** Worcestershire sauce
- **1 lb** fish fillet (tilapia, flounder, cod)
- **48 oz** fish stock
- **1 Tbsp** dry sherry (optional)

1. Place enough olive oil to cover the bottom of an 8-quart soup pot. Add the onion, celery, carrot, and potatoes. Cook on medium heat 5 minutes, stirring occasionally to prevent sticking.

2. Add garlic, basil, oregano, salt, and pepper. Give a quick stir to heat and release aroma of herbs. Cook 1 minute.

3. Add tomatoes, bell pepper, Worcestershire, fish, and fish stock. Simmer 10–15 minutes. Season with salt and pepper.

4. Soup can be finished with a splash of sherry, which guests can add as desired.

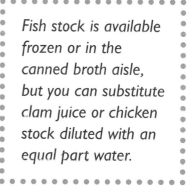

## Cook's Tip

*Fish stock is available frozen or in the canned broth aisle, but you can substitute clam juice or chicken stock diluted with an equal part water.*

**EXCHANGES/CHOICES:** 1/2 STARCH, 2 VEGETABLE, 2 LEAN MEAT
CALORIES 190, CALORIES FROM FAT 40,
TOTAL FAT 4.5 G, SATURATED FAT 1.1 G, TRANS FAT 0 G,
CHOLESTEROL 40 MG, SODIUM 595 MG, TOTAL CARBOHYDRATE 21 G,
DIETARY FIBER 3 G, SUGARS 7 G, PROTEIN 18 G

*This refreshing* **Mango Tuna Salad** *has a surprise crunch from the jicama, while the mango adds its own sweetness and lots of Vitamin C.*

**Serves 4 / Serving Size: 1/4 recipe**

# mango tuna salad

- **4 oz** plain low-fat yogurt
- **6 oz** chunk white or albacore tuna in spring water
- **2 Tbsp** finely minced red onion
- **1 cup** jicama
- **1** large mango, diced into 1/4-inch pieces (additional for garnish)
- **1/2 cup** roughly chopped cilantro (additional for garnish)
- **1** lime, juiced
- **1/4 tsp** fine sea salt
- **1/8 tsp** freshly ground pepper
- **4 cups** mixed greens, washed and dried
- **1/2 cup** toasted sunflower or pumpkin seeds (for garnish)

1. Drain yogurt through a cheesecloth or coffee filter placed in a strainer that has been placed in a bowl to reduce whey and make a thicker consistency.

2. Mix tuna, red onion, jicama, mango, cilantro, lime juice, and half the yogurt. Blend well. Add remaining yogurt as necessary for desired consistency. Add salt and pepper to taste.

3. Serve over mixed greens and garnish with additional mango, sunflower seeds, and cilantro.

### Cook's Tip

*Leftover jicama makes a great addition to any salad or a great dipper for the Basil Pesto Cream on page 139.*

**EXCHANGES/CHOICES: 1 STARCH, 1 VEGETABLE, 2 LEAN MEAT, 1 FAT**
**CALORIES 220, CALORIES FROM FAT 80,**
**TOTAL FAT 9 G, SATURATED FAT 1.2 G, TRANS FAT 0 G,**
**CHOLESTEROL 20 MG, SODIUM 215 MG, TOTAL CARBOHYDRATE 23 G,**
**DIETARY FIBER 5 G, SUGARS 13 G, PROTEIN 15 G**

*This **Mediterranean Fish Stew** is one of those dishes that are packed full of flavor and good-for-you ingredients.*

**Serves 4 / Serving Size: 1/4 recipe**

# mediterranean fish stew

**1** medium to large zucchini

**1** medium eggplant

**1/2 tsp** fine sea salt

**2 (10 oz) cans** chickpeas, drained and rinsed

**2 Tbsp** extra virgin olive oil

**3 cloves** garlic, minced

**2 tsp** Italian seasoning

**3** bay leaves

**1 (28 oz) can** no-salt-added diced tomatoes

**1/4 tsp** freshly grated black pepper

**1 lb** thick white fillet (cod, halibut, or large tilapia)

1. Thinly slice zucchini into rounds and set aside. Cut eggplant into similar sized pieces. Place eggplant in a bowl and sprinkle with 1/2 tsp salt. Toss well. Drain chickpeas in a colander and rinse well.

2. Place the olive oil in the skillet. Add garlic and eggplant and cook until they begin to soften. Clear a space in the bottom of the pan and add the Italian seasoning and bay leaves. Cook 1 minute until the seasonings become fragrant.

3. Add zucchini, chickpeas, tomatoes, and pepper. Mix well. Top with fish, cover, and cook for 10 minutes.

## Cook's Tip

*Rinsing and draining canned beans helps to remove any preservatives and some of the gas. Remove the bay leaves before serving. They are sharp and can cause injury if swallowed.*

**EXCHANGES/CHOICES:** 1 1/2 STARCH, 3 VEGETABLE, 3 LEAN MEAT, 1 FAT
CALORIES 390, CALORIES FROM FAT 90,
TOTAL FAT 10 G, SATURATED FAT 1.4 G, TRANS FAT 0 G,
CHOLESTEROL 50 MG, SODIUM 555 MG, TOTAL CARBOHYDRATE 46 G,
DIETARY FIBER 12 G, SUGARS 14 G, PROTEIN 31 G

*Adding fish to chili is a great way to add more fish to your diet. This **Mixed Bean Chili with Cod** is great for those who are not fish lovers.*

**Serves 8 / Serving Size: 1/8 recipe**

# mixed bean chili with cod

- **1 tsp** canola oil
- **1 1/2 cups** onion, chopped
- **2** large green bell peppers, chopped
- **2** celery stalks, sliced 1/2-inch thick
- **2** large carrots, sliced 1/2-inch thick
- **3 cloves** garlic, minced
- **1 Tbsp** jalapeño pepper, seeded and minced (optional)
- **1/8 tsp** cayenne pepper
- **2 tsp** cumin
- **1/8 tsp** ground cloves
- **2 tsp** dried oregano
- **8 cups** assorted canned beans, rinsed and drained
- **8 cups** canned diced tomatoes
- **1/2 cup** chopped cilantro or Italian parsley
- **1 lb** cod or any mild fish fillet
- **1/3 cup** grated low-fat cheddar cheese (for garnish)
- **1 bunch** scallions, sliced (for garnish)

1. Heat the oil in a large soup pot over medium-high heat. Add the onion, peppers, celery, and carrots and sauté until onion is translucent. Stir in the garlic, jalapeño, cayenne, cumin, cloves, and oregano. Sauté 2–3 minutes.

2. Add the beans, tomatoes, and cilantro (or parsley) and bring to a boil. Reduce heat and simmer, covered, for 30 minutes or more to allow flavors to blend. Add the cod and cook 10 minutes.

3. Garnish each serving with cilantro, cheese, and scallions.

**Cook's Tip**

*Wear rubber gloves when seeding and chopping the jalapeño pepper.*

**EXCHANGES/CHOICES: 2 1/2 STARCH, 3 VEGETABLE, 3 LEAN MEAT**
**CALORIES 400, CALORIES FROM FAT 40,**
**TOTAL FAT 4.5 G, SATURATED FAT 0.9 G, TRANS FAT 0 G,**
**CHOLESTEROL 30 MG, SODIUM 390 MG, TOTAL CARBOHYDRATE 63 G,**
**DIETARY FIBER 17 G, SUGARS 14 G, PROTEIN 30 G**

*These beautiful **Radicchio & Shrimp Salad Cups** make an impressive and colorful first course or light lunch.*

**Serves 4 / Serving Size: 1/4 recipe**

# radicchio & shrimp salad cups

**1 head** radicchio

**8 oz** small, cooked, peeled, and deveined shrimp

**1 tsp** extra virgin olive oil

**2 tsp** white balsamic vinegar

**1/8 tsp** fine sea salt

**1/8 tsp** ground black pepper

**2 Tbsp** fresh pomegranate seeds

**2 Tbsp** chopped fresh parsley

1. Separate radicchio leaves. Reserve eight of the largest.

2. In a large bowl, mix shrimp, olive oil, vinegar, salt, pepper, pomegranate seeds, and parsley. Set aside.

3. Place pairs of radicchio leaves together to form four cups. Fill with equal amounts of shrimp salad.

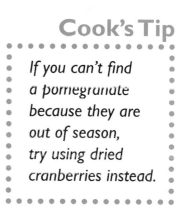

## Cook's Tip

*If you can't find a pomegranate because they are out of season, try using dried cranberries instead.*

EXCHANGES/CHOICES: 1 LEAN MEAT, 1/2 FAT
CALORIES 65, CALORIES FROM FAT 15,
TOTAL FAT 1.5 G, SATURATED FAT 0.3 G, TRANS FAT 0 G,
CHOLESTEROL 90 MG, SODIUM 180 MG, TOTAL CARBOHYDRATE 3 G,
DIETARY FIBER 1 G, SUGARS 1 G, PROTEIN 10 G

*After you've tried it, you'll want something this tasty with every meal.*
*This Shrimp Frisee & Orange Salad is great with leftover*
*sliced meats, such as filet mignon or roasted chicken.*

**Serves 4 / Serving Size: 1/4 recipe, 4 Tbsp dressing**

# shrimp frisee & orange salad

**1/4 cup** pignoli (pine nuts), toasted
**1 large bulb** fennel, sliced on mandolin
**2 cups** baby spinach
**1 medium head** frisee or green leaf lettuce
**1/4 cup** crumbled Gorgonzola cheese

**olive oil and balsamic vinegar dressing**
**1/4 cup** balsamic vinegar
**1/2 cup** extra virgin olive oil
**1 drop** orange oil or orange extract

**1 (11 oz) can** Mandarin oranges, drained
**1 lb** medium, frozen, cooked, peeled, and deveined shrimp

1. Toast nuts by placing them in a small dry skillet and cooking until golden. Remove from pan and cool.

2. Wash and dry salad ingredients. Place in large salad bowl. Top with crumbled Gorgonzola cheese and toasted pignoli.

3. Place vinegar in medium-size bowl. Slowly whisk in olive oil until mixture has been emulsified to a creamy texture. Add orange oil.

4. Add olive oil and balsamic vinegar dressing to greens in small amounts and toss well. Add oranges and shrimp and toss gently.

## Cook's Tip

*Salad should not be swimming in dressing. It's better to add less and decide you need more.*

EXCHANGES/CHOICES: 1/2 FRUIT, 1 VEGETABLE, 2 LEAN MEAT, 3 FAT
CALORIES 285, CALORIES FROM FAT 160,
TOTAL FAT 18 G, SATURATED FAT 3.3 G, TRANS FAT 0 G,
CHOLESTEROL 135 MG, SODIUM 330 MG, TOTAL CARBOHYDRATE 13 G,
DIETARY FIBER 4 G, SUGARS 6 G, PROTEIN 19 G

*Make this* Tortellini Soup with Seafood Medley *on a moment's notice. It can be on the table in 30 minutes or less.*

**Serves 8 / Serving Size: 1/8 recipe**

# tortellini soup with seafood medley

**1 Tbsp** extra virgin olive oil

**2 cloves** garlic, minced

**32 oz** no-salt-added chicken stock

**32 oz** no-salt-added vegetable stock

**28 oz** no-salt-added diced tomatoes

**12 oz** water

**1 cup** fresh basil, chopped

**1/2 cup** fresh oregano, roughly chopped

**2 cups** baby spinach

**10 oz** cheese tortellini

**10 oz** sliced fresh cremini mushrooms

**1 (16 oz) bag** frozen seafood medley

1. Heat olive oil and garlic in soup pot over medium heat until garlic is fragrant.

2. Add chicken and vegetable stock, tomatoes, and water. Bring to a boil.

3. Add basil, oregano, spinach, tortellini, and mushrooms. Cook until tortellini is almost done, approximately 6 minutes. Add seafood medley and cook for 3 minutes more. More water or stock can be added to achieve desired consistency.

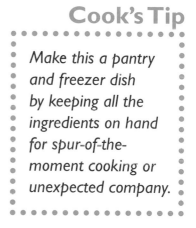

## Cook's Tip

*Make this a pantry and freezer dish by keeping all the ingredients on hand for spur-of-the-moment cooking or unexpected company.*

EXCHANGES/CHOICES: 1 STARCH, 2 VEGETABLE, 2 LEAN MEAT
CALORIES 225, CALORIES FROM FAT 55,
TOTAL FAT 6 G, SATURATED FAT 1.8 G, TRANS FAT 0 G,
CHOLESTEROL 110 MG, SODIUM 440 MG, TOTAL CARBOHYDRATE 26 G,
DIETARY FIBER 3 G, SUGARS 6 G, PROTEIN 18 G

*Washing a large variety of greens at once will make it easier to include a green salad with each meal. This **Tre Colore Salad with Vinaigrette** is a fabulous example of how to fit more greens into your meal plan.*

**Serves 12 / Serving Size: I cup greens, I Tbsp dressing**

# tre colore salad with vinaigrette

**1 head** green leaf lettuce
**1 small head** radicchio
**1 medium head** Belgian endive
**1 half** pomegranate, seeds only
**1 Tbsp** Basic Vinaigrette (recipe on page **138**)

1. Wash and dry salad ingredients. Tear and place in large salad bowl.

2. Add Basic Vinaigrette (recipe on page **138**) in small amounts and toss well.

## Cook's Tip

*Salad should not be swimming in dressing. It's better to add less and decide you need more. Drying greens in a salad spinner helps the dressing cling to the greens.*

EXCHANGES/CHOICES: 2 FAT
CALORIES 100, CALORIES FROM FAT 80,
TOTAL FAT 9 G, SATURATED FAT 1.2 G, TRANS FAT 0 G,
CHOLESTEROL 0 MG, SODIUM 25 MG, TOTAL CARBOHYDRATE 4 G,
DIETARY FIBER 1 G, SUGARS 2 G, PROTEIN 1 G

*This **Tuna and Edamame Salad** recipe takes a delicious new twist on a classic tuna and white bean salad.*

**Serves 4 / Serving Size: 1/4 recipe**

# tuna and edamame salad

**16 oz** edamame (about 2 cups)

**2 Tbsp** orange juice

**1/2 tsp** light soy sauce

**1 tsp** rice wine vinegar

**1/2 tsp** freshly ground pepper (divided use)

**2 Tbsp, plus 1 tsp** extra virgin olive oil (divided use)

**4 cloves** garlic, sliced (about 2 Tbsp)

**16 oz** tuna steak, cut into 4 portions

**1/4 tsp** fine sea salt

**1** orange, sliced (for garnish)

1. Place edamame in medium mixing bowl. Add orange juice, soy sauce, rice wine vinegar, and 1/4 tsp pepper to the edamame. Mix well. Set aside to allow flavors to blend.

2. Place 2 Tbsp extra virgin olive oil in small saucepan. Add garlic and heat to medium. Cook until garlic begins to turn golden brown. Add to the bowl with the edamame.

3. Brush tuna with 1 tsp extra virgin olive oil and season with sea salt and 1/4 tsp pepper. Heat grill pan. Grill tuna lightly on each side.

4. Serve tuna topped with the edamame salad. Garnish with orange slices.

## Cook's Tip

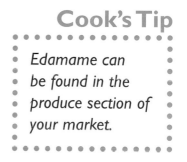

*Edamame can be found in the produce section of your market.*

EXCHANGES/CHOICES: 1 CARBOHYDRATE, 5 LEAN MEAT, 2 FAT
CALORIES 390, CALORIES FROM FAT 170,
TOTAL FAT 19 G, SATURATED FAT 3.1 G, TRANS FAT 0 G,
CHOLESTEROL 40 MG, SODIUM 220 MG, TOTAL CARBOHYDRATE 18 G,
DIETARY FIBER 7 G, SUGARS 7 G, PROTEIN 38 G

*This **Warm Shrimp and Bean Salad** is so quick and easy you won't believe you can create such wonderful flavor in such a short time. It is great with whole-grain Italian bread.*

**Serves 6 / Serving Size: 1/6 recipe**

# warm shrimp and bean salad

**1/4 cup** extra virgin olive oil

**6 cloves** garlic, thinly sliced lengthwise

**1 head** broccoli, cut into florets (about 2 1/2 cups)

**1/2 cup** chicken stock or dry white wine (Orvieto or Pinot Grigio)

**1 lb** large shrimp, peeled and deveined

**2 cups** small white beans, drained and rinsed (15–16 oz can)

**1 cup** diced fresh roma tomatoes (3 large tomatoes)

**1/4 tsp** fine sea salt

**1/4 tsp** freshly ground pepper

1. Place olive oil in small saucepan. Heat and then add sliced garlic. Watch carefully and cook until golden. Remove garlic from oil with slotted spoon and drain on paper towels. Cool and reserve oil. You will use 1 Tbsp in this recipe and store the remainder for later use. Store the extra oil in a clean, dry bottle at room temperature.

2. Place 1 Tbsp garlic oil in sauté pan. Add broccoli and sauté 2–3 minutes. Add chicken stock. Cover and cook 5 minutes.

3. Add shrimp and white beans. Cover and cook approximately 5 minutes until shrimp turn pink and are opaque inside.

4. Add tomatoes, salt, and pepper. Toss well. Garnish with toasted garlic.

EXCHANGES/CHOICES: 1 STARCH, 2 LEAN MEAT
CALORIES 170, CALORIES FROM FAT 30,
TOTAL FAT 3.5 G, SATURATED FAT 0.5 G, TRANS FAT 0 G,
CHOLESTEROL 85 MG, SODIUM 420 MG, TOTAL CARBOHYDRATE 20 G,
DIETARY FIBER 5 G, SUGARS 3 G, PROTEIN 16 G

*Seafood Sausage is usually lightly seasoned, but when you use it in a dish like this* **White Bean Soup**, *it becomes much more flavorful.*

**Serves 8 / Serving Size: 1/8 recipe**

# white bean soup

**1 Tbsp** extra virgin olive oil

**2 cups** diced onion

**4 large cloves** garlic, minced

**1 cup** carrot, cut into 1/2-inch-thick slices

**1 cup** celery, cut into 1/2-inch-thick slices

**3 cans (15 oz each)** small white beans, drained and rinsed

**2 quarts** no-salt-added chicken stock

**2 quarts** water

**2** bay leaves

**1/4 tsp** fine sea salt

**1/4 tsp** freshly ground pepper

**1 (6 oz) bag** baby spinach

**1 lb** seafood sausage (from the seafood counter of your favorite gourmet market)

1. Thinly film an 8-quart soup pot with oil. Add onion, garlic, carrots, and celery and cook until vegetables begin to brown.

2. Add beans, stock, water, bay leaves, salt, and pepper. Cook at least 1 hour. Add spinach and seafood sausage and cook another 10 minutes until sausage is cooked and spinach is limp.

## Cook's Tip

*Any variety of Italian-style sausage will work for a change of pace with this dish.*

EXCHANGES/CHOICES: 1 1/2 STARCH, 1 VEGETABLE, 2 LEAN MEAT, 1 FAT
CALORIES 285, CALORIES FROM FAT 70,
TOTAL FAT 8 G, SATURATED FAT 1.4 G, TRANS FAT 0 G,
CHOLESTEROL 30 MG, SODIUM 575 MG, TOTAL CARBOHYDRATE 32 G,
DIETARY FIBER 7 G, SUGARS 5 G, PROTEIN 23 G

# Chapter 3:

# SALMON

*This **Asian Stuffed Salmon Fillet** was inspired by something a friend prepared, and I am so glad she introduced me to the idea.*

**Serves 8 / Serving Size: 1/8 recipe**

# asian stuffed salmon fillet

**1 Tbsp** canola oil

**3** baby bok choy, julienned

**1 (6 oz) bag** baby spinach

**2 cups** fresh bean sprouts
   (about 1/2 lb)

**10 oz** fresh mushrooms, sliced

**2** carrots, shredded

**3** scallions, sliced thinly

**2 inches** ginger, peeled and grated
   or finely minced

**2 cloves** garlic, minced

**1/4 cup** light soy sauce

**2 lb** salmon fillet, skin removed

**1/4 cup** mild honey

**1/4 cup** Dijon mustard

1. Preheat oven to 450°.

2. Pour canola oil in sauté pan. Add all vegetables, ginger, and garlic. Cook until tender but firm. Add soy sauce and cook an additional 5 minutes. Remove from pan and spread on a large baking sheet to cool slightly.

3. Place salmon on a large sheet of heavy-duty aluminum foil. Cut salmon through center lengthwise. Remove top piece. Cover bottom half with vegetables. Top with the remaining piece of salmon fillet.

4. Mix honey and mustard. Brush fish with honey mustard. Wrap fish in foil. Place on baking sheet and bake until fish is flaky, about 20 minutes. Slice into 8 portions.

**Cook's Tip**

*1 inch of fresh ginger is approximately 1 Tbsp of grated or minced ginger.*

**EXCHANGES/CHOICES:** 1/2 **CARBOHYDRATE,** 2 **VEGETABLE,** 4 **LEAN MEAT**
**CALORIES** 285, **CALORIES FROM FAT** 110,
**TOTAL FAT** 12 G, **SATURATED FAT** 1.9 G, **TRANS FAT** 0 G,
**CHOLESTEROL** 75 MG, **SODIUM** 565 MG, **TOTAL CARBOHYDRATE** 17 G,
**DIETARY FIBER** 3 G, **SUGARS** 13 G, **PROTEIN** 28 G

*I love one-pot meals and the blend of flavors in this **Balsamic Salmon on Barley Pilaf** dish makes it extra special.*

**Serves 4 / Serving Size: 1/4 recipe**

# balsamic salmon on barley pilaf

- **1 Tbsp** canola oil
- **1** medium onion, finely chopped
- **1 large clove** garlic, finely minced
- **2 stalks** celery, thinly sliced (about 2 cups)
- **4** carrots, thinly sliced (about 1 1/2 cups)
- **1 cup** barley, uncooked

- **3 cups** low-sodium chicken stock
- **1 pint** cherry tomatoes, cut in half
- **1/4 cup** balsamic vinegar
- **1/2 cup** basil leaves, roughly chopped
- **1/4 tsp** fine sea salt
- **1/8 tsp** freshly ground black pepper
- **1 lb** salmon fillet, skin removed, cut into 4 pieces (4 oz each)

1. Place canola oil in large stockpot. Heat and add onion, garlic, and celery. Cook over medium heat, covered, until onion becomes translucent. Add carrots and barley and cook uncovered until barley begins to look toasted. Add stock. Cover and cook 30 minutes.

2. Slice tomatoes in half and place in large bowl with balsamic vinegar, basil, salt, pepper, and salmon. Let this sit while the barley is cooking for the first 30 minutes. After 30 minutes, remove salmon from tomato mixture. Stir tomato mixture into barley and place salmon on top of barley. Cover and cook 10 minutes more to steam the salmon.

3. Place some barley pilaf in a pasta bowl and top with a piece of salmon to serve.

## Cook's Tip

*Cherry and grape tomatoes are always in season. I like to buy them each time I shop so I have them on hand at all times for a quick burst of color, flavor, and nutrition.*

**EXCHANGES/CHOICES:** 2 1/2 STARCH, 3 VEGETABLE, 3 LEAN MEAT, 1 FAT
**CALORIES** 440, **CALORIES FROM FAT** 110,
**TOTAL FAT** 12 G, **SATURATED FAT** 2.1 G, **TRANS FAT** 0 G,
**CHOLESTEROL** 55 MG, **SODIUM** 350 MG, **TOTAL CARBOHYDRATE** 51 G,
**DIETARY FIBER** 12 G, **SUGARS** 9 G, **PROTEIN** 34 G

*The bourbon sauce in this **Cedar Plank Salmon with Bourbon** dish really complements the flavor imparted from the cedar plank.*

**Serves 4 / Serving Size: 1/4 recipe**

# cedar plank salmon with bourbon

**1** food-grade cedar plank
**1 Tbsp** canola oil
**1 cup** chopped onion (about 1 large)
**2 cloves** garlic, peeled and minced
**1 (15 oz) can** petite diced tomatoes
**1 cup** chicken stock
**1 Tbsp** Worcestershire sauce
**1/4 cup** bourbon
**1/4 tsp** freshly ground black pepper
**1** large onion, sliced 1/4-inch thick
**1 lb** salmon fillet, with skin

1. Preheat oven to 400°. Soak cedar plank in water for at least 20 minutes while preparing bourbon sauce. This will prevent charring.

2. Place canola oil in medium saucepan. Add chopped onion and cook until it begins to brown. Add garlic and cook until garlic becomes fragrant, about 1 minute. Add tomatoes, stock, Worcestershire sauce, bourbon, and pepper. Bring to a boil, reduce heat, and simmer 20 minutes.

3. In the meantime, remove cedar plank from water and place on large baking sheet. Spread sliced onion on plank. Place salmon fillet, skin side down, on top of onions. Brush top of salmon lightly with 2 Tbsp of bourbon sauce. Bake 25–30 minutes until fish is cooked completely.

4. Serve with cedar plank onions and additional bourbon sauce on the side.

EXCHANGES/CHOICES: 3 VEGETABLE, 3 LEAN MEAT, 2 FAT
CALORIES 305, CALORIES FROM FAT 125,
TOTAL FAT 14 G, SATURATED FAT 2 G, TRANS FAT 0 G,
CHOLESTEROL 75 MG, SODIUM 550 MG, TOTAL CARBOHYDRATE 16 G,
DIETARY FIBER 2 G, SUGARS 8 G, PROTEIN 27 G

*It would be great if every dish had the same satisfying crunchiness
as this **Crispy Salmon with Lemon Dill Sauce** recipe.*

**Serves 6 / Serving Size: 1/6 recipe**

# crispy salmon with lemon dill sauce

**8 oz** low-fat plain yogurt

**1/2 cup** snipped dill

**2** lemons, juiced (divided use)

**3** egg whites

**2 tsp** cornstarch

**1 cup** bread crumbs

**2** lemons, zested

**1/2 tsp** salt

**1 Tbsp** canola oil

**1 lb** salmon fillet, skin removed, cut into 6 pieces

1. Mix yogurt, dill, and juice of 1 lemon together in small bowl.
   Set aside. Mix juice of 1 lemon, egg whites, and cornstarch
   in another shallow bowl. Mix bread crumbs, lemon zest,
   and salt in a third bowl.

2. Dip salmon in egg white mixture, then in bread crumbs. Set
   aside on large dinner plate until all pieces are coated.

3. Place canola oil in nonstick sauté pan. Heat pan and slowly
   add salmon. Brown on all sides and serve with lemon dill
   sauce.

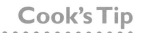

## Cook's Tip

*It would be ok to zest
the lemons first, and
then use them for the
juice in this dish. Or
you can store a "zested"
lemon in a plastic bag in
the fridge for later use.*

**EXCHANGES/CHOICES:** 1 STARCH, 3 LEAN MEAT, 1/2 FAT
CALORIES 240, CALORIES FROM FAT 70,
TOTAL FAT 8 G, SATURATED FAT 1.7 G, TRANS FAT 0 G,
CHOLESTEROL 55 MG, SODIUM 420 MG, TOTAL CARBOHYDRATE 18 G,
DIETARY FIBER 1 G, SUGARS 4 G, PROTEIN 22 G

*Lovely to look at and as fresh as summer itself,* **Grilled Salmon & Asparagus** *can be served hot or cold. Serve it with a baguette or pasta.*

**Serves 4 / Serving Size: 1/4 recipe**

# grilled salmon & asparagus

**2 Tbsp** extra virgin olive oil

**2 cloves** garlic, chopped

**1/4 cup** fresh basil leaves, thinly sliced

**2** lemons, juiced

**1 lb** thick salmon fillet, skinless, cut into 4 portions

**2 tsp** salt-free lemon pepper seasoning

**2 lb** thin asparagus, ends broken off and placed in a bowl of water

1. Place olive oil in small sauté pan. Add garlic and heat until garlic becomes fragrant, about 2 minutes. Add basil and turn heat off. Whisk in lemon juice. Set aside.

2. Sprinkle salmon with lemon pepper seasoning. Set aside.

3. Preheat grill pan for a few minutes. Drain asparagus and place on grill pan. Cover and roast asparagus for 3 minutes, shaking occasionally. Remove cover. Brush salmon with lemon garlic bath. Place on the grill pan. Cook first side until a nice crust forms. Turn and cook second side. If you want your salmon well done, the lid can be placed on the grill pan.

4. Place asparagus on serving plate. Top with salmon. Drizzle with lemon garlic bath. Additional lemon garlic bath can be stored for future use.

## Cook's Tip

*The asparagus with the garlic bath would make a nice side dish for any grilled protein source.*

EXCHANGES/CHOICES: 2 VEGETABLE, 4 LEAN MEAT, 2 FAT
CALORIES 300, CALORIES FROM FAT 155,
TOTAL FAT 17 G, SATURATED FAT 2.6 G, TRANS FAT 0 G,
CHOLESTEROL 75 MG, SODIUM 80 MG, TOTAL CARBOHYDRATE 9 G,
DIETARY FIBER 3 G, SUGARS 3 G, PROTEIN 29 G

*Celery Root is a very fresh tasting vegetable that complements the flavor of this* **Grilled Salmon Steak with Celery Root and Parsley**.

**Serves 4 / Serving Size: 1/4 recipe**

# grilled salmon steak
## with celery root and parsley

**4** salmon steaks (about 4 oz each)

**1 tsp** extra virgin olive oil

**1 Tbsp** balsamic vinegar

**1 lb** celery root

**1/2 cup** chopped Italian parsley (additional for garnish, if desired)

**1/4 tsp** fine sea salt

**1/8 tsp** freshly ground black pepper

1. Place salmon in 9-inch square baking dish. Mix olive oil and balsamic vinegar together. Pour over salmon steaks. Set aside for 20 minutes.

2. Peel celery root and cut into 1-inch cubes. Place in 4-quart saucepan and cover with water (about 3 cups). Bring to a boil and cook until celery root is fork tender, about 15 minutes. Drain and mash. Stir in the parsley, salt, and pepper. Keep warm (yields about 2 cups).

3. Preheat grill pan. Remove salmon from marinade and drain well. Grill on medium about 4 minutes per side.

4. Serve a salmon steak with 1/2 cup celery root and parsley mixture. Garnish with additional chopped parsley.

## Cook's Tip

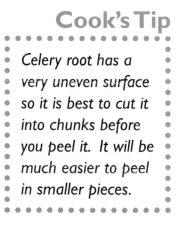

*Celery root has a very uneven surface so it is best to cut it into chunks before you peel it. It will be much easier to peel in smaller pieces.*

EXCHANGES/CHOICES: 1 VEGETABLE, 3 LEAN MEAT, 1 FAT
CALORIES 225, CALORIES FROM FAT 90,
TOTAL FAT 10 G, SATURATED FAT 1.8 G, TRANS FAT 0 G,
CHOLESTEROL 75 MG, SODIUM 270 MG, TOTAL CARBOHYDRATE 7 G,
DIETARY FIBER 1 G, SUGARS 1 G, PROTEIN 25 G

*Kale is a super vitamin-packed green that many of us don't use often enough. It complements the ingredients in this* **Grilled Salmon Steak with Kale and Sun-Dried Tomatoes** *recipe perfectly.*

**Serves 4 / Serving Size: 1/4 recipe**

# grilled salmon steak
## with kale and sun-dried tomatoes

**16 oz** kale, washed and cut

**1 Tbsp** extra virgin olive oil

**1** small onion, chopped (1/2 cup)

**1 clove** garlic, crushed, peeled, and minced

**1/2 cup** chopped sun-dried tomatoes (not in oil)

**4** salmon steaks (about 4 oz each)

**1/4 tsp** fine sea salt

**1/4 tsp** freshly ground black pepper

**1/4 cup** balsamic vinegar

**2 Tbsp** pignoli (pine nuts), toasted

1. Place kale in large colander and rinse. Shake excess water from greens. Set aside.

2. Place olive oil and onion in large skillet. Heat and cook until onion becomes golden brown. Add greens, garlic, and sun-dried tomatoes. Cook until greens are wilted and tender. They will cook down substantially. If pan becomes too dry, add water as necessary.

3. While greens are cooking, preheat grill pan. Sprinkle salmon steaks on both sides with salt and pepper. Grill 3 minutes on each side.

4. Place nuts in dry skillet and cook until golden brown. Remove immediately from skillet so that they do not burn.

5. Place greens on plate and top with a salmon steak. Sprinkle each serving with balsamic vinegar and pine nuts.

EXCHANGES/CHOICES: 3 VEGETABLE, 3 LEAN MEAT, 1 1/2 FAT
CALORIES 325, CALORIES FROM FAT 155,
TOTAL FAT 17 G, SATURATED FAT 2.5 G, TRANS FAT 0 G,
CHOLESTEROL 75 MG, SODIUM 235 MG, TOTAL CARBOHYDRATE 17 G,
DIETARY FIBER 4 G, SUGARS 7 G, PROTEIN 28 G

*Mediterranean flavors are my absolute favorite and this delicious* **Lemony Poached Salmon with a Fennel, Onion & Olive Salad** *recipe is a great example of why.*

**Serves 4 / Serving Size: 1/4 recipe**

# lemony poached salmon
## with a fennel, onion & olive salad

**1 lb** salmon fillet, skin removed, cut into 4 portions
**1** lemon, juiced
Water to cover salmon

**salad**
**1/2 cup** thinly sliced fennel tops
**1/2** medium red onion, thinly sliced
**1/2 cup** pitted olives
**1/2 cup** sliced cucumber

**4 cups** red leaf lettuce, washed, dried, and torn into bite-sized pieces
**1** lemon, sliced for garnish

**dressing**
**1** lemon, juiced
**2 Tbsp** extra virgin olive oil
**1/4 tsp** fine sea salt
**1/4 tsp** black pepper
**1 Tbsp** capers

1. Prepare pan for poaching. Place salmon in pan. Add lemon juice and enough water to cover. Bring to a boil. Lower heat and simmer for 5–7 minutes, or until it flakes with a fork.

2. Place salad ingredients in large bowl.

3. Whisk lemon juice, oil, salt, and pepper together. Add capers. Pour half of the dressing over the salad greens. Toss. Save the rest of the dressing to use with another salad.

4. Place salad on plate and top with salmon. Garnish with additional lemon slices.

EXCHANGES/CHOICES: 1 VEGETABLE, 3 LEAN MEAT, 1 1/2 FAT
CALORIES 230, CALORIES FROM FAT 110,
TOTAL FAT 12 G, SATURATED FAT 2.1 G, TRANS FAT 0 G,
CHOLESTEROL 50 MG, SODIUM 310 MG, TOTAL CARBOHYDRATE 6 G,
DIETARY FIBER 2 G, SUGARS 2 G, PROTEIN 25 G

*Cooking with fruit is a refreshing change. The fruits in this **Pan-Seared Salmon with Strawberry-Kiwi Relish** are available year-round.*

**Serves 8 / Serving Size: 1/4 cup**

# pan-seared salmon
## with strawberry-kiwi relish

**1 lb** salmon fillet, skin removed, cut into 4 pieces
**1 tsp** wasabi mustard

---

### strawberry-kiwi relish

**1 pint** strawberries, washed and sliced
**2** kiwis, peeled and diced
**1/4 cup** cilantro, roughly chopped
**1** orange, juiced

1. Coat salmon with wasabi mustard. Set aside.

2. Mix together strawberries, kiwis, cilantro, and orange juice in a large mixing bowl. Set aside to allow flavors to blend.

3. Heat large nonstick sauté pan. Add salmon and sear on all sides until nicely browned.

4. Place a large spoonful of strawberry-kiwi relish on a plate and place salmon on top. Garnish with fresh cilantro sprigs.

5. Serve with brown rice or couscous.

## Cook's Tip

*For a change of pace, replace the kiwi with a another fruit, such as Mandarin oranges.*

EXCHANGES/CHOICES: 1 FRUIT, 3 LEAN MEAT, 1 FAT
CALORIES 255, CALORIES FROM FAT 90,
TOTAL FAT 10 G, SATURATED FAT 1.7 G, TRANS FAT 0 G,
CHOLESTEROL 75 MG, SODIUM 75 MG, TOTAL CARBOHYDRATE 15 G,
DIETARY FIBER 3 G, SUGARS 10 G, PROTEIN 25 G

*This **Roasted Salmon with Vegetables** recipe is a delightful blend of fresh, delicious, and good-for-you ingredients.*

**Serves 4 / Serving Size: 1/4 recipe**

# roasted salmon with vegetables

**1 lb** fennel, quartered and thinly sliced (about 4 cups)

**1 lb** zucchini, quartered and thinly sliced (about 4 cups)

**1 lb** eggplant, cut into 1-inch cubes (about 4 cups)

**6 cloves** garlic, peeled

**1 tsp** fine sea salt

**1 Tbsp** extra virgin olive oil

**1/4 tsp** black pepper

**1 tsp** Italian seasoning blend

**1 lb** salmon fillet with skin

1. Preheat oven to 400°.

2. Place vegetables in large bowl with salt. Toss well. (This will draw moisture out of them and create a barrier so they will not absorb more oil than necessary.) Let sit 10 minutes. Add oil, pepper, and Italian seasoning to bowl and toss well.

3. Line a baking sheet with parchment paper. Place vegetables on parchment in single layer. Roast vegetables 10 minutes.

4. Dip salmon in reserved vegetable bowl to absorb any leftover juices from the vegetables. Place salmon, skin side up, in the center of the vegetables. Roast for 20 minutes.

5. Remove skin from salmon and cut into 4 portions. Place some vegetables on a plate and top with a piece of the salmon.

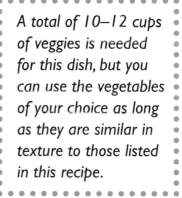

**Cook's Tip**

*A total of 10–12 cups of veggies is needed for this dish, but you can use the vegetables of your choice as long as they are similar in texture to those listed in this recipe.*

**EXCHANGES/CHOICES: 3 VEGETABLE, 3 LEAN MEAT, 2 FAT**
**CALORIES 305, CALORIES FROM FAT 125,**
**TOTAL FAT 14 G, SATURATED FAT 2.2 G, TRANS FAT 0 G,**
**CHOLESTEROL 75 MG, SODIUM 705 MG, TOTAL CARBOHYDRATE 19 G,**
**DIETARY FIBER 6 G, SUGARS 6 G, PROTEIN 28 G**

*When you need a change of pace in the kitchen, try a new cooking method.*
*Kids will enjoy making these **Salmon & Couscous Packages**.*

**Serves 4 / Serving Size: 1/4 recipe**

# salmon & couscous packages

**4 pieces** heavy-duty aluminum foil

Cooking spray

**1/4** cup fresh dill, minced

**5 Tbsp** nonfat sour cream (divided use)

**1 lb** salmon fillet, skin removed, cut into 4 pieces

**1 cup** uncooked couscous

**2 cups** dry white wine or vermouth

**1/4 tsp** fine sea salt

**1/8 tsp** black pepper

**1** cucumber, washed, unpeeled, and sliced 1/4-inch thick

1. Preheat oven to 400°.

2. Tear off four pieces of aluminum foil large enough to hold one piece of salmon each. Spray with cooking spray. Lift edges of foil to prevent liquid from spilling.

3. Mix dill and 4 Tbsp of sour cream. Spread sour cream mixture on salmon.

4. Sprinkle 1/4 cup couscous in center of each piece of foil. Place salmon on top. Pour 1/2 cup white wine into each package. Sprinkle with salt and black pepper. Gather up corners of foil and tightly close packages. Place on baking sheet and bake for 15 minutes.

5. Toss sliced cucumbers with sour cream and let sit while fish cooks. Serve with cucumbers and sour cream.

EXCHANGES/CHOICES: 2 1/2 STARCH, 4 LEAN MEAT, 1/2 FAT
CALORIES 405, CALORIES FROM FAT 90,
TOTAL FAT 10 G, SATURATED FAT 1.7 G, TRANS FAT 0 G,
CHOLESTEROL 80 MG, SODIUM 75 MG, TOTAL CARBOHYDRATE 36 G,
DIETARY FIBER 2 G, SUGARS 3 G, PROTEIN 31 G

*This **Salmon & Spinach Pie** recipe is like a quiche but lighter, with health benefits from the spinach, salmon, and tofu.*

**Serves 8 / Serving Size: 1/8 recipe**

# salmon & spinach pie

**14 oz** light firm tofu, drained
Cooking spray
**2 Tbsp** Italian-style bread crumbs
**1 Tbsp** canola oil
**1** small onion, chopped (1/2 cup)
**9 oz** fresh spinach (about 8 cups)
**4 oz** salmon fillet, skin removed, chopped

**4** egg whites
**2 tsp** Deliciously Dill Salt-Free Seasoning
**1/4 tsp** salt
**1/4 tsp** black pepper
**2 oz** light havarti cheese, shredded

1. Preheat oven to 375°. Place rack in center of oven.

2. Break tofu into small pieces and place in colander to drain further.

3. Spray 8" pie plate with cooking spray. Sprinkle with bread crumbs and set aside.

4. Place canola oil in nonstick sauté pan. Add onion and cook until onion becomes translucent. Add spinach and cover. Cook until spinach cooks down. Add salmon and cook just until salmon is pink. Set aside.

5. Place egg whites, dill, salt, and pepper in large mixing bowl. Add tofu. Mix well by hand. Add spinach mixture. Mix well. Place in prepared pie plate. Top with grated cheese. Bake 30 minutes or until top is golden and center is set. Cool 10 minutes for easier cutting and neater slices.

### Cook's Tip

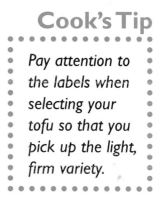

*Pay attention to the labels when selecting your tofu so that you pick up the light, firm variety.*

EXCHANGES/CHOICES: 1/2 CARBOHYDRATE, 1 MEDIUM-FAT MEAT
CALORIES 115, CALORIES FROM FAT 45,
TOTAL FAT 5 G, SATURATED FAT 1.2 G, TRANS FAT 0 G,
CHOLESTEROL 10 MG, SODIUM 225 MG, TOTAL CARBOHYDRATE 5 G,
DIETARY FIBER 1 G, SUGARS 1 G, PROTEIN 12 G

*The added spice of chili paste and red pepper really complements the salmon in this colorful **Salmon Chili Stir-Fry** dish.*

**Serves 4 / Serving Size: 1/4 recipe**

# salmon chili stir-fry

- **1 tsp** Thai red chili paste
- **1/2 cup** low-sodium chicken stock
- **1 lb** salmon fillet, skin removed, cut into thin strips
- **1 tsp** canola oil
- **4 oz** snow peas (1 cup), sliced in half lengthwise
- **1 bunch** scallions, cut in half vertically and in half again horizontally
- **1 cup** matchstick carrots
- **1** red bell pepper, seeded and cut into julienned strips
- **10 oz** canned baby corn, cut in half vertically
- **2 Tbsp** stir-fry ginger seasoning

1. Mix chili paste with chicken stock. Place salmon in a dish large enough to hold it in a single layer. Pour chili mixture over salmon. Let salmon marinate while doing the preparation for the rest of the ingredients.

2. Place canola oil in large nonstick sauté pan. Add vegetables and stir-fry and cook to desired tenderness. Push vegetables to the side and add salmon. Stir-fry until opaque. Add stir-fry ginger seasoning and mix salmon, vegetables, and season well.

3. Serve with brown rice.

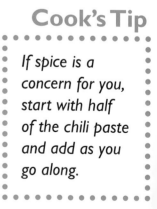

## Cook's Tip

*If spice is a concern for you, start with half of the chili paste and add as you go along.*

**EXCHANGES/CHOICES: 2 VEGETABLE, 3 LEAN MEAT, 1 1/2 FAT**
**CALORIES 255, CALORIES FROM FAT 100,**
**TOTAL FAT 11 G, SATURATED FAT 1.9 G, TRANS FAT 0 G,**
**CHOLESTEROL 75 MG, SODIUM 95 MG, TOTAL CARBOHYDRATE 12 G,**
**DIETARY FIBER 4 G, SUGARS 6 G, PROTEIN 27 G**

*I have been asked for a fish taco recipe many times. I think these* **Salmon**

**Tacos** *are great with the addition of mango, arugula, and avocado.*

**Serves 4 / Serving Size: I taco**
# salmon tacos

**1/2 lb** salmon fillet, skin removed, cut into 1/4-inch strips

**1 tsp** salt-free Mexican seasoning

**1/2** Haas avocado, peeled and cut into 1/4-inch strips

**1 cup** diced mango

**2 cups** fresh arugula

**8 tsp** canned tomatoes and green chilis

**4** corn taco shells

1. Sprinkle salmon with Mexican seasoning. Sauté salmon in nonstick skillet for 3–5 minutes or until cooked thoroughly.

2. Fill each taco shell with 1/4 of all ingredients.

## Cook's Tip

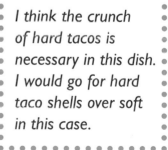

*I think the crunch of hard tacos is necessary in this dish. I would go for hard taco shells over soft in this case.*

**EXCHANGES/CHOICES:** 1/2 STARCH, 1/2 FRUIT, 2 LEAN MEAT, 1 1/2 FAT
CALORIES 225, CALORIES FROM FAT 100,
TOTAL FAT 11 G, SATURATED FAT 1.8 G, TRANS FAT 0 G,
CHOLESTEROL 40 MG, SODIUM 215 MG, TOTAL CARBOHYDRATE 19 G,
DIETARY FIBER 4 G, SUGARS 7 G, PROTEIN 14 G

*This **Salmon with Black Bean Salsa** is so beautiful you will want to make it all the time. The colors are exquisite and it takes very little time to prepare.*

**Serves 4 / Serving Size: 1/4 recipe**

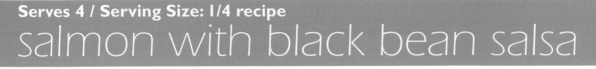

# salmon with black bean salsa

**2 tsp** soy sauce

**1 Tbsp** orange juice

**1 lb** thick salmon fillet, skin removed, cut into 4 pieces

**black bean salsa**

**15 oz** black beans, drained and rinsed

**1** soft mango, diced

**1/2 tsp** ground cumin

**1 Tbsp** extra virgin olive oil

**1/2 cup** chopped cilantro

**2** fresh limes, juiced

**2 Tbsp** minced red onion

**1/8 tsp** fine sea salt

**1/8 tsp** freshly ground pepper

1. Mix soy sauce and orange juice in plastic bag. Add salmon and marinate for at least 20 minutes and up to 2 hours.

2. Mix black bean salsa ingredients together in large bowl. (Prepare salsa early in the day to allow flavors to blend.)

3. Preheat grill or grill pan. Add salmon and grill until nicely browned.

4. Place 1/2 cup black bean salsa on plate and place salmon on top. Garnish with fresh cilantro sprigs (if desired).

## Cook's Tip

*Leftover salsa can be tossed into a green salad the next day.*

**EXCHANGES/CHOICES: 1/2 STARCH, 1/2 FRUIT, 4 LEAN MEAT, 1 FAT**
**CALORIES 295, CALORIES FROM FAT 110,**
**TOTAL FAT 12 G, SATURATED FAT 2.1 G, TRANS FAT 0 G,**
**CHOLESTEROL 75 MG, SODIUM 360 MG, TOTAL CARBOHYDRATE 18 G,**
**DIETARY FIBER 4 G, SUGARS 8 G, PROTEIN 28 G**

*When I think of all the recipes in this book, this* Salmon with a Sweet Potato Crust *is one of my favorites because it has a spicy and flavorful crunch with added coolness from the sauce.*

**Serves 4 / Serving Size: 1/4 recipe**

# salmon with sweet potato crust

**cucumber cilantro sauce**
**8 oz** low-fat yogurt
**1/2 cup** cucumber, diced
**1/4 cup** chopped cilantro

---

**2** eggs whites
**1/2 cup** all-purpose flour
**1 1/2 cups** shredded sweet potato (about 1/2 lb)
**1 lb** salmon fillet, skin removed, cut into 4 portions
**2 tsp** garam masala no-salt spice blend
**2 tsp** canola oil

1. Mix ingredients for cucumber cilantro sauce and set aside.

2. Place egg whites, flour, and sweet potatoes in three separate small bowls.

3. Rinse salmon. Sprinkle with garam masala. Dip salmon in egg, then flour, then egg, and finally sweet potato.

4. Place canola oil in large nonstick sauté pan and heat. Add fish and brown all sides until golden.

5. Serve with cucumber cilantro sauce.

## Cook's Tip

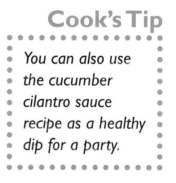

*You can also use the cucumber cilantro sauce recipe as a healthy dip for a party.*

**EXCHANGES/CHOICES:** 1 1/2 STARCH, 4 LEAN MEAT, 1 FAT
CALORIES 345, CALORIES FROM FAT 115,
TOTAL FAT 13 G, SATURATED FAT 2.5 G, TRANS FAT 0 G,
CHOLESTEROL 80 MG, SODIUM 130 MG, TOTAL CARBOHYDRATE 24 G,
DIETARY FIBER 2 G, SUGARS 7 G, PROTEIN 31 G

*This* **Savory Salmon Baked in a Crisp Crust** *is an elegant and show-stopping entree that will have your guests raving.*

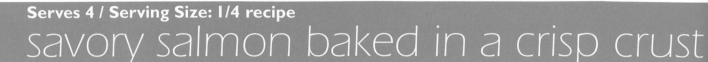

**Serves 4 / Serving Size: 1/4 recipe**

# savory salmon baked in a crisp crust

**8 oz** low-fat plain yogurt
**3** scallions, thinly sliced
**1/4 cup** minced fresh dill
**20 sheets** (each 9″ × 14″) phyllo dough (defrosted in refrigerator for 3 hours or more)
Cooking spray
**1 lb** salmon fillet, skin removed, cut into 4 portions
**4 Tbsp** honey mustard

1. Preheat oven to 375°.

2. Mix yogurt with scallions and dill. Set aside.

3. Open phyllo and lay flat on counter. Cover with a damp tea towel to keep it from drying out. Take 1 leaf of phyllo and lay it on the work surface. Spray with cooking spray. Repeat until you have 5 layers.

4. Brush each piece of salmon with 1 Tbsp honey mustard and spoon yogurt mixture on top. Lay 1 piece of salmon in center of each piece of phyllo. Sprinkle with freshly ground black pepper.

5. Fold each side of phyllo over salmon. Turn ends under salmon to prevent bottom from getting soggy. Spray outside of each package with cooking spray. Place on baking sheet and bake for 30 minutes.

6. Serve with steamed broccoli with lemon juice, salt, and pepper.

### Cook's Tip

*Never defrost phyllo in a microwave...it would be way too hot to handle.*

**EXCHANGES/CHOICES: 3 STARCH, 4 LEAN MEAT, 1/2 FAT**
**CALORIES 425, CALORIES FROM FAT 115,**
**TOTAL FAT 13 G, SATURATED FAT 2.3 G, TRANS FAT 0 G,**
**CHOLESTEROL 80 MG, SODIUM 415 MG, TOTAL CARBOHYDRATE 45 G,**
**DIETARY FIBER 2 G, SUGARS 8 G, PROTEIN 34 G**

# Chapter 4:

# TUNA, SWORDFISH & HALIBUT

*For something a little different or for those who are not fond of fish, this **Baked Swordfish with Horseradish** recipe is the one to try. Your taste buds will focus on the horseradish crust.*

**Serves 4 / Serving Size: 1/4 recipe**

# baked swordfish with horseradish

**1/2 cup** prepared horseradish (squeeze dry)

**2** scallions, finely chopped

**1/4 tsp** wasabi powder

**1/4 tsp** ground ginger

**1/4 tsp** Dijon mustard

**1/4 tsp** lemon zest

**1/2 cup** unseasoned bread crumbs

**1 tsp** finely chopped shallot

**1/4 cup** fresh lemon juice

**1 Tbsp** extra virgin olive oil

**16 oz** swordfish, cut into 4 portions

**1/2 cup** white wine

1. Preheat oven to 475°.

2. Place all ingredients, except wine and fish, in food processor. Blend evenly.

3. Place swordfish in 9 × 13-inch baking dish. Pat horseradish mixture on top. Pour wine over top. Bake at 475° for about 20 minutes.

## Cook's Tip

*This recipe works well with any thick fish steak or even a boneless, skinless chicken breast.*

EXCHANGES/CHOICES: 1/2 STARCH, 1 VEGETABLE, 3 LEAN MEAT, 1 FAT
CALORIES 250, CALORIES FROM FAT 80,
TOTAL FAT 9 G, SATURATED FAT 1.9 G, TRANS FAT 0 G,
CHOLESTEROL 45 MG, SODIUM 305 MG, TOTAL CARBOHYDRATE 15 G,
DIETARY FIBER 2 G, SUGARS 4 G, PROTEIN 25 G

*The veggies in this* **Chili Garlic Tuna with Peanut-Sauced Veggies** *dish are a great alternative to rice or noodles.*

**Serves 4 / Serving Size: 1/4 recipe**

# chili garlic tuna
## with peanut-sauced veggies

**16 oz** tuna steak, cut into 4 portions

**2 Tbsp** chili garlic paste

**2 tsp** canola oil

**1** medium onion, diced (about 1 cup)

**2 cups** matchstick carrots

**9 oz** baby spinach (1 large bag)

**1 can** diced water chestnuts (about 8 oz)

**2 cups** broth

**2 Tbsp** peanut sauce (found in Asian section
of your supermarket)

1. Cut tuna into 2 × 2 squares and place in ceramic dish. Mix with chili garlic paste. Preheat grill pan for 5 minutes. Add tuna and cook 3 minutes on each side.

2. Place canola oil in large sauté pan. Heat to medium and add onions, carrots, spinach, and water chestnuts. Sauté until spinach wilts. Add broth and peanut sauce and toss. Cook until carrots are tender.

3. Serve tuna with vegetable mixture.

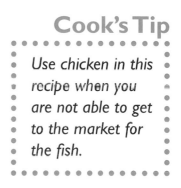

## Cook's Tip

*Use chicken in this recipe when you are not able to get to the market for the fish.*

**EXCHANGES/CHOICES: 3 VEGETABLE, 3 LEAN MEAT, 1 FAT**
**CALORIES 270, CALORIES FROM FAT 80,**
**TOTAL FAT 9 G, SATURATED FAT 1.7 G, TRANS FAT 0 G,**
**CHOLESTEROL 45 MG, SODIUM 790 MG, TOTAL CARBOHYDRATE 18 G,**
**DIETARY FIBER 5 G, SUGARS 7 G, PROTEIN 30 G**

*Cocoa and pepper are a "hot" combo right now. Some of the finest chocolatiers are working with different kinds of pepper and chocolate combinations. This* **Cocoa Pepper Halibut** *is subtle but sublime.*

**Serves 2 / Serving Size: 1/2 recipe**

# cocoa pepper halibut

**cocoa pepper rub**

**1 Tbsp** paprika

**2 Tbsp** freshly ground black pepper

**1 Tbsp** onion powder

**1 tsp** cocoa powder

**1/2 tsp** cayenne pepper

**1/2 tsp** Splenda

**16 oz** halibut steak

**2 tsp** canola oil

**1/4 cup** white wine or stock

1. Mix all ingredients together for cocoa pepper rub. Rub halibut with a few drops of canola oil and then cocoa rub. Discard any extra cocoa rub that has been exposed to fish.

2. Place remaining canola oil in a nonstick pan and heat to medium. Cook halibut for 2 minutes on first side. Turn. Add stock, cover, and cook 8 minutes more.

**Cook's Tip**

*I used halibut in this dish; however, any mild steak fish will work for this recipe.*

EXCHANGES/CHOICES: 1/2 CARBOHYDRATE, 7 LEAN MEAT
CALORIES 330, CALORIES FROM FAT 90,
TOTAL FAT 10 G, SATURATED FAT 1.2 G, TRANS FAT 0 G,
CHOLESTEROL 70 MG, SODIUM 130 MG, TOTAL CARBOHYDRATE 7 G,
DIETARY FIBER 2 G, SUGARS 2 G, PROTEIN 48 G

*Halloumi is a cheese from Cypress that is brined and browns well when cooked. I used it in this Greek-Style Swordfish as it gives the flavor that you get from olives, but also the crunch from the browning.*

**Serves 4 / Serving Size: 1/4 recipe**

# greek-style swordfish

**3 oz** Halloumi light cheese, broken up into large "crumbles"

**16 oz** swordfish steak, cut into 1-inch cubes

**1/2 cup** chopped sun-dried tomatoes (not in oil)

**3 Tbsp** capers

**2** lemons, juiced

**2 tsp** Greek seasoning

**2** medium zucchini, quartered and sliced 1/4-inch thick (about 2 cups)

**1 1/3 cups** cooked brown rice.

1. In a large nonstick skillet, sauté the Halloumi for 8–10 minutes until it begins to turn golden brown.

2. Add the swordfish and cook an additional 3–5 minutes or until fish begins to brown. Add sun-dried tomatoes, capers, lemon juice, Greek seasoning, and zucchini. Cook until zucchini is tender.

3. Serve with 1/3 cup brown rice per serving.

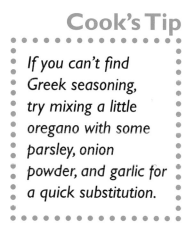

**Cook's Tip**

*If you can't find Greek seasoning, try mixing a little oregano with some parsley, onion powder, and garlic for a quick substitution.*

EXCHANGES/CHOICES: 1 STARCH, 1 VEGETABLE, 4 LEAN MEAT, 1/2 FAT
CALORIES 295, CALORIES FROM FAT 80,
TOTAL FAT 9 G, SATURATED FAT 3.5 G, TRANS FAT 0 G,
CHOLESTEROL 50 MG, SODIUM 450 MG, TOTAL CARBOHYDRATE 25 G,
DIETARY FIBER 4 G, SUGARS 5 G, PROTEIN 32 G

*This **Grilled Swordfish with Lentils & Fig Vincotto** has two great flavor components that make it exceptional. Vincotto is bursting with flavor, while the Parmigiano garnish really finishes this dish nicely.*

**Serves 4 / Serving Size: 1/4 recipe**

# grilled swordfish
## with lentils & fig vincotto

3 **Tbsp** extra virgin olive oil (divided use)
1 medium onion, chopped (about 1 cup)
2 **cloves** garlic, peeled and minced (about 1 Tbsp)
3 medium carrots, halved and thinly sliced (about 1 cup)
2 **stalks** celery, halved and thinly sliced (about 1 cup)
1 **cup** dried lentils (small Italian or French lentils preferred)

4 **cups** low-sodium, fat-free chicken or vegetable stock
1/4 **tsp** salt
1/4 **tsp** black pepper
1 **cup** fresh basil, chopped
16 **oz** swordfish steak, cut into 4 portions
2 **Tbsp** freshly grated Parmigiano-Reggiano
2 **Tbsp** fig vincotto

1. Place 2 Tbsp olive oil in a 5-quart saucepan. Add the onion and garlic and cook on medium heat until the onion begins to brown. Add carrots, celery, and lentils and toss. Turn pan to high and add 2 cups stock. Once it comes to a boil, turn to simmer and cook until most of the stock is evaporated, about 10 minutes. Add remaining stock and cook until tender. The total cooking time will be about 25–30 minutes. Stir in salt, pepper, and basil.

2. During the last 10–15 minutes of cooking time, preheat grill pan. Brush swordfish with remaining olive oil and place on hot grill pan. Cook 4 minutes on first side, turn, and continue to cook until desired doneness.

3. Place 1/4 of the vegetable mixture in a soup plate and top with 1/4 of the fish, Pamigiano-Reggiano, and fig vincotto.

EXCHANGES/CHOICES: 2 STARCH, 5 LEAN MEAT, 1 1/2 FAT
CALORIES 440, CALORIES FROM FAT 145,
TOTAL FAT 16 G, SATURATED FAT 3.1 G, TRANS FAT 0 G,
CHOLESTEROL 45 MG, SODIUM 295 MG, TOTAL CARBOHYDRATE 38 G,
DIETARY FIBER 13 G, SUGARS 8 G, PROTEIN 37 G

*The basil cream in this **Grilled Tuna with Basil Cream** dish also makes a flavorful and healthy low-fat dip or spread for veggies or low-fat chips. Your guests will not believe it is so good for them!*

**Serves 4 / Serving Size: 1/4 recipe**

# grilled tuna with basil cream

- **1 cup** fresh baby spinach
- **2 cloves** garlic, minced
- **1** large shallot, quartered
- **1/4 cup** grated Parmigiano-Reggiano
- **1/2 cup** fresh basil
- **1 cup** nonfat cottage cheese
- **2 tsp** extra virgin olive oil
- **16 oz** fresh tuna steak, cut into 4 portions
- **1/4 tsp** fine sea salt
- **1/4 tsp** fresh black pepper

1. Place spinach, garlic, shallot, Parmigiano-Reggiano, and basil in a food processor. Process until finely minced. With the motor running, add cottage cheese. Process until smooth. Set aside.

2. Preheat grill pan. Rub tuna with oil, salt, and pepper. Place on grill and cook first side 4–5 minutes. Turn and cook other side to desired doneness.

3. Serve with basil cream mixture.

## Cook's Tip

*Basil cream can be made a day or two ahead of time. Leftover basil cream can be used as a dip, spread, or tossed with pasta.*

**EXCHANGES/CHOICES: 4 LEAN MEAT**
**CALORIES 190, CALORIES FROM FAT 70,**
**TOTAL FAT 8 G, SATURATED FAT 1.8 G, TRANS FAT 0 G,**
**CHOLESTEROL 45 MG, SODIUM 240 MG, TOTAL CARBOHYDRATE 1 G,**
**DIETARY FIBER 0 G, SUGARS 0 G, PROTEIN 27 G**

*This **Grilled Tuna with Garlic Aioli & Baby Greens on Crusty Rolls** is, by far, one of my favorite ways to enjoy a tuna steak. It is a perfect combination of flavors and ingredients, just like a good BLT.*

**Serves 4 / Serving Size: 1/4 recipe**

# grilled tuna with garlic aioli
## & baby greens on crusty rolls

**2 cloves** garlic, grated (about 1 Tbsp)

**1/4 cup** light mayonnaise

**2 cups** mixed baby greens

**12 oz** tuna steak, cut into 4 portions, about 1/4 inch-thick

**1 tsp** extra virgin olive oil

**1/8 tsp** fine sea salt

**1/8 tsp** freshly ground pepper

**4** Portuguese or hard rolls (2 oz each)

1. Mince garlic with a grater or zester. Stir into mayo. Set aside. Wash and dry salad greens in salad spinner.

2. Place tuna in a large shallow dish and season with olive oil, salt, and pepper. Heat grill pan. Grill tuna lightly on each side.

3. Cut rolls in half vertically. Layer tuna, 1 Tbsp aioli, and greens. Top with other half of the roll.

## Cook's Tip

*A pouched tuna steak would also work well if you don't want to grill fresh tuna.*

**EXCHANGES/CHOICES:** 2 STARCH, 3 LEAN MEAT, 1 FAT
**CALORIES** 345, **CALORIES FROM FAT** 110,
**TOTAL FAT** 12 G, **SATURATED FAT** 2.3 G, **TRANS FAT** 0 G,
**CHOLESTEROL** 35 MG, **SODIUM** 545 MG, **TOTAL CARBOHYDRATE** 32 G,
**DIETARY FIBER** 2 G, **SUGARS** 3 G, **PROTEIN** 25 G

*Osso Buco is one of my very favorite dishes and this Halibut in the Style of Osso Buco dish is fantastic. The bone-in halibut steak is reminiscent of the classic veal shank preparation.*

**Serves 4 / Serving Size: 1/4 recipe**

# halibut in the style of osso buco

**1 cup** sliced carrots

**1 cup** sliced celery

**1/2 cup** chopped onion

**1/2 cup** Wondra flour

**1/2 tsp** fine sea salt

**1/4 tsp** freshly ground black pepper

**1 Tbsp** extra virgin olive oil

**16 oz** halibut steak with bone

**4 cloves** garlic

**1/2 cup** chopped fresh basil

**2 Tbsp** chopped fresh marjoram or oregano

**1 cup** dry white wine or vermouth

**1 cup** clam juice or chicken stock

**1 (14.5 oz) can** diced tomatoes

**1** lemon, zested

**2 cloves** minced garlic (divided use)

**1/2 cup** finely minced Italian parsley

1. Place carrots, celery, and onion in food processor with steel blade. Pulse until finely minced.

2. Place flour in large bowl or pie plate. Season with salt and pepper. Place just enough olive oil in pan to lightly coat bottom. Heat oil. While oil is heating, dredge fish in flour. Brown fish on both sides, about 4 minutes on each side.

3. Remove fish from pan. Add carrots, celery, 1 clove garlic, and onion. Sauté 5 minutes and add basil and marjoram. Add wine, clam juice (or stock), and tomatoes. Bring to boil. Lower heat and return fish to pan. Cover and simmer for 15 minutes. Grate zest of lemon, 1 clove minced garlic, and parsley. Mix together and reserve for garnish.

4. Serve this dish over polenta, small pasta, risotto, or mashed potatoes with plenty of the sauce.

EXCHANGES/CHOICES: 1/2 STARCH, 3 VEGETABLE, 2 LEAN MEAT, 1/2 FAT
CALORIES 245, CALORIES FROM FAT 55,
TOTAL FAT 6 G, SATURATED FAT 0.8 G, TRANS FAT 0 G,
CHOLESTEROL 30 MG, SODIUM 660 MG, TOTAL CARBOHYDRATE 22 G,
DIETARY FIBER 4 G, SUGARS 6 G, PROTEIN 23 G

*This delightful **Halibut with Garlicky Vegetable Trio**
recipe is as colorful as it is quick, delicious, and nutritious.*

**Serves 4 / Serving Size: 1/4 recipe**

# halibut with garlicky vegetable trio

**1/2 cup** Wondra flour

**1/2 tsp** fine sea salt

**1/4 tsp** freshly ground pepper

**16 oz** halibut steak, cut into 4 portions

**1 Tbsp** extra virgin olive oil

**2 cloves** garlic, minced

**1/2 cup** white wine or chicken stock

**1/2 cup** chicken stock

**2 cups** baby carrots, sliced lengthwise

**1** red bell pepper, sliced into 1/4-inch strips

**1/2 lb** fresh green beans, stemmed

**1/2 cup** flat Italian parsley, roughly chopped (divided use)

1. Mix flour, salt, and pepper in shallow bowl. Dredge fish in flour and set aside.

2. Place olive oil in large sauté pan and turn heat to medium. Add fish. Brown fish 2–3 minutes on each side or until golden. Add garlic and cook until fragrant, about 1 minute.

3. Add the wine and chicken stock to deglaze pan. Add the vegetables and 1/4 cup parsley. Cover and simmer 5 minutes to steam vegetables. Garnish with remaining parsley.

4. Serve over small pasta, rice, or couscous.

## Cook's Tip

*Wondra, commonly known as instant flour, is a fine granular flour that is also used to make smooth sauces. All-purpose flour can be substituted.*

**EXCHANGES/CHOICES: 1/2 STARCH, 3 VEGETABLE, 3 LEAN MEAT, 1/2 FAT
CALORIES 270, CALORIES FROM FAT 65,
TOTAL FAT 7 G, SATURATED FAT 1.0 G, TRANS FAT 0 G,
CHOLESTEROL 35 MG, SODIUM 380 MG, TOTAL CARBOHYDRATE 23 G,
DIETARY FIBER 5 G, SUGARS 6 G, PROTEIN 28 G**

*En papillote means that you are baking in parchment paper or aluminum foil. Each person gets their own little dinner present to open with this Herbed Tuna En Papillote.*

**Serves 4 / Serving Size: I package**

# herbed tuna en papillote

Parchment paper
**10 oz** frozen artichoke hearts, defrosted slightly
**16 oz** tuna steak, cut into 4 portions
**4 sprigs** fresh basil
**4 Tbsp** sun-dried tomatoes
**4 cloves** garlic, peeled and minced
**1/8 tsp** fine sea salt
**1/8 tsp** freshly ground pepper
**1/4 cup** dry white vermouth

1. Preheat oven to 425°.

2. Cut four sheets of parchment paper, about 18" long, and fold in half. Cut each into a heart shape.

3. Working in the center of each parchment heart, layer as follows: artichoke hearts, I piece fish, 3–4 leaves fresh basil, I Tbsp sun-dried tomatoes, I clove garlic, pinch of salt, a few grinds of black pepper, and I Tbsp vermouth.

4. Fold the parchment hearts in half and begin to crimp the edges, making a tight seal. You will end up with a little tail at the end. Tuck the tail under the parchment and place on the baking sheet. Bake 15 minutes until parchment is lightly browned and puffed. Place a parchment package on each of 4 dinner plates and allow each diner to open their "present."

**EXCHANGES/CHOICES: 2 VEGETABLE, 3 LEAN MEAT**
**CALORIES 205, CALORIES FROM FAT 55,**
**TOTAL FAT 6 G, SATURATED FAT 1.4 G, TRANS FAT 0 G,**
**CHOLESTEROL 40 MG, SODIUM 115 MG, TOTAL CARBOHYDRATE 9 G,**
**DIETARY FIBER 3 G, SUGARS 2 G, PROTEIN 28 G**

*This **Involtini Di Pesce Spaca** dish means "stuffed swordfish in the Siciliian style" and is inspired by a cooking class I took in Siena, Italy.*

**Serves 4 / Serving Size: 1/4 recipe**

# involtini di pesce spada

**1 cup** plain, dry bread crumbs
**1/4 tsp** fine sea salt
**1/4 tsp** chili pepper or crushed red pepper flakes
**2 cloves** garlic, minced (divided use)
**1/2 cup** raisins or dried mixed fruit bits
**1/4 cup** pignoli (pine nuts)
**2 cups** fresh basil leaves, chopped (divided use)
**3/4 cup** dry white wine (divided use)
**1 lb** swordfish, sliced very thin (2–4 slices, depending on thickness)
**1 cup** plum tomatoes, diced (about 2 large)
**1 tsp** extra virgin olive oil

1. Preheat oven to 375°.

2. Mix together the bread crumbs, salt, chili pepper, 1 clove garlic, raisins, 1/8 cup pignoli, 1 cup basil, and 1/2 the wine. Cover swordfish with 1/2 cup of the stuffing and roll into wraps. Tie with kitchen twine.

3. Place tomatoes, olive oil, and remaining basil and white wine in a 9 × 9 casserole dish large enough to hold the involtini. Lay the fish on top of this mixture. Turn fish and coat outside with this mixture. Finish seam side down.

4. Bake for 25–30 minutes. Slice fish into pinwheels and top with sauce. Serve with sautéed baby spinach with pignoli, crushed red pepper, and 1 clove garlic.

**EXCHANGES/CHOICES: 1 STARCH, 1 FRUIT, 1 VEGETABLE, 3 LEAN MEAT**
**CALORIES 395, CALORIES FROM FAT 115,**
**TOTAL FAT 13 G, SATURATED FAT 2.1 G, TRANS FAT 0 G,**
**CHOLESTEROL 45 MG, SODIUM 455 MG, TOTAL CARBOHYDRATE 38 G,**
**DIETARY FIBER 4 G, SUGARS 15 G, PROTEIN 29 G**

*The sweet and spice of this **Key Lime Swordfish with Apple Radish Salad** recipe will please even the pickiest palate.*

**Serves 4 / Serving Size: 1/4 recipe**

# key lime swordfish
## with apple radish salad

**1 lb** swordfish steak, cut into 4 portions

**2 tsp** Key lime pepper blend

### apple radish salad

**1** Granny Smith apple, diced (about 1 1/2 cups)

**3 stalks** celery, thinly sliced (about 1 cup)

**1 Tbsp** extra virgin olive oil

**1/2 cup** chopped fresh cilantro (additional for garnish)

**2** limes, juiced

**1 (6 oz) bag** radishes, sliced (about 1 1/2 cups)

**2 Tbsp** canned, diced green chilies

**1/4 tsp** fine sea salt

**1/4 tsp** freshly ground black pepper

1. Sprinkle swordfish with Key lime pepper blend. Heat grill pan. Add swordfish and grill on each side for 4 minutes.

2. While swordfish is cooking, mix all ingredients of the apple radish salad together in a medium bowl and set aside.

3. Place a piece of swordfish on each plate with 1 cup apple radish salad. Garnish with fresh cilantro sprigs.

## Cook's Tip

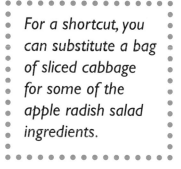

*For a shortcut, you can substitute a bag of sliced cabbage for some of the apple radish salad ingredients.*

EXCHANGES/CHOICES: 1/2 STARCH, 1 VEGETABLE, 3 LEAN MEAT, 1/2 FAT
CALORIES 210, CALORIES FROM FAT 70,
TOTAL FAT 8 G, SATURATED FAT 1.7 G, TRANS FAT 0 G,
CHOLESTEROL 45 MG, SODIUM 305 MG, TOTAL CARBOHYDRATE 11 G,
DIETARY FIBER 3 G, SUGARS 7 G, PROTEIN 23 G

This **Roasted Citrus Garlic Swordfish** *is so colorful and filled with flavor, you'll want to make it all the time.*

**Serves 4 / Serving Size: 1/4 recipe**

# roasted citrus garlic swordfish

**3** leeks, thinly sliced (about 2 cups)
**1** medium zucchini, halved and thinly sliced (1 1/2 cups)
**1** medium yellow squash, halved and thinly sliced (1 1/2 cups)
**1 cup** grape tomatoes
**2 large cloves** garlic, crushed and peeled
**1 Tbsp, plus 1 tsp** extra virgin olive oil (divided use)
**1/2 tsp** fine sea salt (divided use)
**1/4 tsp** freshly ground black pepper
**16 oz** swordfish steak, cut into 4 portions
**1 tsp** extra virgin olive oil

1. Preheat oven to 400°.

2. Rinse leeks well. Drain and place in a large bowl. Add zucchini, yellow squash, tomatoes, garlic, 1 Tbsp extra virgin olive oil, 1/4 tsp salt, and pepper. Toss well. Spread in an 8 × 10 baking dish.

3. Rub fish with remaining 1 tsp olive oil and 1/4 tsp salt. Place fish on top of the vegetables.

4. Place baking dish in center of oven and roast for 35 minutes, turning fish after 15 minutes.

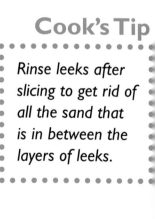

## Cook's Tip

*Rinse leeks after slicing to get rid of all the sand that is in between the layers of leeks.*

EXCHANGES/CHOICES: 2 VEGETABLE, 3 LEAN MEAT, 1 FAT
CALORIES 230, CALORIES FROM FAT 80,
TOTAL FAT 9 G, SATURATED FAT 1.9 G, TRANS FAT 0 G,
CHOLESTEROL 45 MG, SODIUM 415 MG, TOTAL CARBOHYDRATE 12 G,
DIETARY FIBER 3 G, SUGARS 5 G, PROTEIN 25 G

*This **Seared Tuna & White Beans** recipe is reminiscent of a dish I first enjoyed in Venice, Italy several years ago.*

**Serves 4 / Serving Size: 1/4 recipe**

# seared tuna & white beans

**4 Tbsp** extra virgin olive oil

**1/2 cup** chopped rosemary leaves

**2 tsp** crushed hot red pepper

**1 clove** garlic, peeled and crushed

**16 oz** tuna steak, cut 2 inches thick

**2 oz** pancetta, finely chopped

**2 cups** white beans, rinsed and drained

**8 medium slices** fresh tomato

1. Heat olive oil in small sauté pan and add rosemary, red pepper, and garlic. Set aside to cool. (This will keep several weeks in a clean, airtight jar.)

2. Heat 1 Tbsp of the infused oil in a large nonstick skillet over medium-high heat. Add the tuna. Partially cover the pan and cook, searing tuna on all sides, about 1 minute per side.

3. In a separate pan, cook the pancetta. Add beans and cook until beans are heated. Place the bean mixture on a serving platter.

4. Cut the tuna into very thin slices. Fan the slices around the beans. Serve with sliced tomatoes.

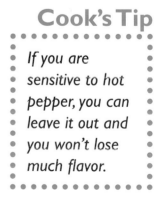

## Cook's Tip

*If you are sensitive to hot pepper, you can leave it out and you won't lose much flavor.*

**EXCHANGES/CHOICES: 1 1/2 STARCH, 5 LEAN MEAT**
**CALORIES 340, CALORIES FROM FAT 100,**
**TOTAL FAT 11 G, SATURATED FAT 2.3 G, TRANS FAT 0 G,**
**CHOLESTEROL 45 MG, SODIUM 385 MG, TOTAL CARBOHYDRATE 26 G,**
**DIETARY FIBER 6 G, SUGARS 3 G, PROTEIN 36 G**

*The combination of tuna and sesame in this Sesame Tuna dish*
*can't be beat and has been proven to be a favorite in many restaurants.*

**Serves 4 / Serving Size: 1/4 recipe**

# sesame tuna

**1** egg white

**1 tsp** soy sauce

**1/2 cup** sesame seeds

**2 tsp** canola oil

**16 oz** tuna steak, cut into 1/4-inch-thick slices

**1 tsp** sugar-free apricot preserves or wasabi
mustard (optional)

1. Place egg white and soy sauce in a small shallow dish. Whisk until well blended. Place sesame seeds in another shallow dish.

2. Dip tuna slices in egg mixture and then in sesame seeds.

3. Heat canola oil in a large nonstick sauté pan. Brown tuna on first side until sesame seeds are golden. Turn and brown second side until sesame seeds are golden.

4. Serve with apricot preserves or wasabi mustard.

## Cook's Tip

*Sautéed Spinach and Garlic (page 155) would also be a nice complement to this recipe.*

EXCHANGES/CHOICES: 4 LEAN MEAT, 2 FAT
CALORIES 285, CALORIES FROM FAT 155,
TOTAL FAT 17 G, SATURATED FAT 2.8 G, TRANS FAT 0 G,
CHOLESTEROL 40 MG, SODIUM 135 MG, TOTAL CARBOHYDRATE 4 G,
DIETARY FIBER 2 G, SUGARS 0 G, PROTEIN 30 G

*This **Swordfish with Chickpeas** recipe was inspired by a friend's description of one of her mother's favorite dishes. I did my best to recreate this delicious dish to do her mother's recipe justice.*

**Serves 4 / Serving Size: 1/4 recipe**

# swordfish with chickpeas

**2 tsp** extra virgin olive oil

**1** medium onion, chopped (about 1 cup)

**3/4 tsp** cumin

**16 oz** swordfish steak, cut into 1-inch cubes or chunks

**2 cloves** garlic, peeled and minced

**1** bay leaf

**1/4 tsp** fine sea salt

**1/4 tsp** freshly ground black pepper

**2 cups** canned chickpeas, drained and rinsed

**2 cups** low-fat, reduced-sodium chicken stock

**1/2 cup** fresh basil, chopped

1. Place olive oil in sauté pan. Turn heat to high and add onion. Sauté onion 2–3 minutes until it begins to brown. Reduce heat if onion is browning too quickly. Add cumin and sauté 1 minute. Add swordfish. Sauté until brown, about 3–5 minutes.

2. Add garlic, bay leaf, salt, and pepper. Sauté 1–2 minutes until seasonings are fragrant.

3. Add chickpeas and stock and simmer 10 minutes. Chickpeas will absorb some of the stock and sauce will reduce slightly.

4. Remove bay leaf and garnish with fresh basil. Serve over couscous grande (the large couscous) with some of the sauce spooned over.

## Cook's Tip

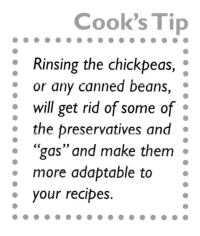

*Rinsing the chickpeas, or any canned beans, will get rid of some of the preservatives and "gas" and make them more adaptable to your recipes.*

**EXCHANGES/CHOICES: 1 STARCH, 1 VEGETABLE, 3 LEAN MEAT, 1 FAT**
**CALORIES 285, CALORIES FROM FAT 80,**
**TOTAL FAT 9 G, SATURATED FAT 1.7 G, TRANS FAT 0 G,**
**CHOLESTEROL 45 MG, SODIUM 610 MG, TOTAL CARBOHYDRATE 23 G,**
**DIETARY FIBER 6 G, SUGARS 5 G, PROTEIN 30 G**

*Spinach is not only healthy, but it is also versatile. It combines beautifully with the sweetness of the apricots and the savory flavor of the swordfish in this **Swordfish with Apricots & Spinach**.*

**Serves 4 / Serving Size: 1/4 recipe**

# swordfish with apricots & spinach

**3** egg whites
**1 cup** Italian-seasoned bread crumbs
**1/4 tsp** fine sea salt
**1/4 tsp** freshly ground black pepper
**1 (9 oz) bag** baby spinach, rinsed (about 8 cups)
**2 tsp** extra virgin olive oil
**16 oz** swordfish steaks
**1 (10 oz) can** apricot halves, drained (juice reserved)

1. Place egg whites in a pie plate. Place bread crumbs in second pie plate and season with salt and pepper to taste.

2. Rinse spinach in colander. Set aside. Cut swordfish into 1-inch strips. Dredge swordfish in egg whites and then bread crumbs.

3. Heat nonstick sauté pan to medium. Add extra virgin olive oil and cook swordfish until crisp and golden on each side. Add apricots, 1/4 cup of the juice, and heat gently.

4. Cook spinach until wilted in a 10- or 12-inch sauté pan. (The spinach will cook in the water that clings to the leaves after rinsing.)

5. Place spinach on a plate and top with fish and apricots.

## Cook's Tip

*Baby spinach is a great refrigerator staple to keep on hand. Check sell-by or use-before dates on the bags for the freshest spinach.*

**EXCHANGES/CHOICES: 1 STARCH, 1 FRUIT, 4 LEAN MEAT**
**CALORIES 305, CALORIES FROM FAT 70,**
**TOTAL FAT 8 G, SATURATED FAT 1.9 G, TRANS FAT 0 G,**
**CHOLESTEROL 45 MG, SODIUM 655 MG, TOTAL CARBOHYDRATE 29 G,**
**DIETARY FIBER 3 G, SUGARS 11 G, PROTEIN 29 G**

*When you are craving something special and creamy, this*
**Tuna with Creamy Cheese Center** *is your go-to dish.*

**Serves 4 / Serving Size: 1/4 recipe**

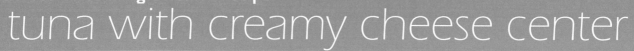

# tuna with creamy cheese center

**2 Tbsp, plus 1 tsp** light herb cheese (Boursin or Alouette)

**1 Tbsp** Wondra flour

**16 oz** tuna steaks (2 steaks at 8 oz each)

**1 tsp** canola oil

**1 cup** low-sodium chicken stock

**4 cups** baby arugula

**4 slices** tomato

1. Divide 2 Tbsp of cheese into 2 balls. Roll into flour.

2. Cut a pocket in each tuna steak and stuff pocket with cheese.

3. Place canola oil in medium nonstick skillet. Heat to medium and add tuna. Brown on first side and turn to brown second side, about 8 minutes total. Once second side is browned, add stock and the remaining 1 tsp of cheese. Blend cheese into sauce. Add arugula and cover. Cook until arugula is wilted.

4. Place tomato slices on plate and top with arugula. Cut tuna steak into two portions and place on top of the tomato slices and arugula. Serve with additional sauce and brown or wild rice.

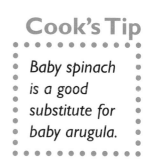

## Cook's Tip

*Baby spinach is a good substitute for baby arugula.*

EXCHANGES/CHOICES: 4 LEAN MEAT
CALORIES 200, CALORIES FROM FAT 70,
TOTAL FAT 8 G, SATURATED FAT 2.1 G, TRANS FAT 0 G,
CHOLESTEROL 45 MG, SODIUM 115 MG, TOTAL CARBOHYDRATE 3 G,
DIETARY FIBER 1 G, SUGARS 1 G, PROTEIN 28 G

*Wasabi peas are great with their spice and crunch and they sing when combined with the orange notes in this **Tuna with Wasabi Crunch & Orange-Scented Baby Bok Choy**.*

**Serves 4 / Serving Size: 1/4 recipe**

# tuna with wasabi crunch
## & orange-scented baby bok choy

**1 cup** wasabi peas

**1/4 tsp** salt

**1 lb** tuna steaks, cut into 4 portions

**1 tsp** hot chili sesame or plain sesame oil

**1 tsp** canola oil

**6** baby bok choy, thinly sliced and rinsed well

**3 oz** fresh orange juice

**1 tsp** light soy sauce

1. Place wasabi peas and salt in food processor fitted with steel blade. Process to a fine cornmeal-like consistency. Press wasabi pea mixture onto fish.

2. Heat both kinds of oil in nonstick sauté pan. Brown fish on one side and turn and brown other side, about 10 minutes total.

3. In the meantime, place rinsed and drained baby bok choy in the second nonstick skillet. Sauté until wilted and add orange juice and soy sauce. Cook another 2 minutes and serve with the tuna.

## Cook's Tip

*I like to purchase sashimi-grade tuna steaks frozen from the store and keep them in my freezer to save me a trip to the store. This is the tuna that they are selling already "defrosted."*

**EXCHANGES/CHOICES: 1 STARCH, 4 LEAN MEAT, 1 FAT
CALORIES 305, CALORIES FROM FAT 100,
TOTAL FAT 11 G, SATURATED FAT 2.9 G, TRANS FAT 0 G,
CHOLESTEROL 40 MG, SODIUM 325 MG, TOTAL CARBOHYDRATE 19 G,
DIETARY FIBER 1 G, SUGARS 6 G, PROTEIN 30 G**

# Chapter 5:

# THIN FILLETS

*Arctic char is a wonderfully sweet, pink-fleshed fish that is a cousin to salmon and trout. This **Arctic Char With Wine & Rosemary** is exceptionally pleasing to those who find salmon a bit strong.*

**Serves 4 / Serving Size: 1/4 recipe**

# arctic char with wine & rosemary

**2 cups** dry white wine (Sauvignon Blanc or Pinot Grigio)
**4 sprigs** fresh rosemary (additional rosemary for garnish, optional)
**1/4 tsp** fine sea salt
**1/4 tsp** freshly ground pepper
**2** fresh lemons, sliced (divided use)
**1 lb** arctic char fillet, skin removed

1. Place wine, rosemary, salt, a few grinds of black pepper, and slices of one lemon in sauté pan.

2. Add fish, bring to low boil, cover, and simmer until fish is done, approximately 10 minutes.

3. Serve with additional lemon slices and sprigs of rosemary.

## Cook's Tip

*You can ask your seafood manager to skin the fish for you.*

EXCHANGES/CHOICES: 4 LEAN MEAT
CALORIES 170, CALORIES FROM FAT 65,
TOTAL FAT 7 G, SATURATED FAT 1.4 G, TRANS FAT 0 G,
CHOLESTEROL 50 MG, SODIUM 85 MG, TOTAL CARBOHYDRATE 0 G,
DIETARY FIBER 0 G, SUGARS 0 G, PROTEIN 24 G

*If you can't visit a tropical island, you can still make this delicious* **Broiled Flounder with Tropical Slaw** *and you'll feel like you're on vacation!*

**Serves 4 / Serving Size: 1/4 recipe**

# broiled flounder with tropical slaw

**1/4 cup** light mayonnaise

**1/4 tsp** ground chipotle pepper

**1 (6 oz) can** crushed pineapple

**1/2 cup** chopped cilantro, or flat Italian parsley

**2 cups** packaged coleslaw mix

Cooking spray

**1 lb** flounder fillet

1. Mix mayonnaise and chipotle pepper together in large bowl. Add pineapple with juice and cilantro. Mix well. Add coleslaw and mix well.

2. Preheat boiler. Spray foil pan with cooking spray and place fish in pan. Spray fish with cooking spray. Place under broiler for 3–5 minutes until fish is flaky.

3. Serve with tropical slaw. This dish can also be served in a whole-wheat pita.

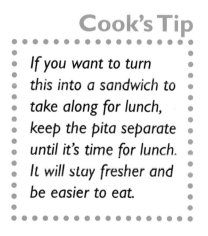

## Cook's Tip

*If you want to turn this into a sandwich to take along for lunch, keep the pita separate until it's time for lunch. It will stay fresher and be easier to eat.*

**EXCHANGES/CHOICES: 1/2 FRUIT, 3 LEAN MEAT, 1/2 FAT**
**CALORIES 180, CALORIES FROM FAT 55,**
**TOTAL FAT 6 G, SATURATED FAT 1.1 G, TRANS FAT 0 G,**
**CHOLESTEROL 65 MG, SODIUM 230 MG, TOTAL CARBOHYDRATE 8 G,**
**DIETARY FIBER 1 G, SUGARS 6 G, PROTEIN 22 G**

*A coulis is simply a thick puree or sauce. This **Broiled Sole with Red Pepper Coulis** is a delicious dish that's fast and super easy to make.*

**Serves 4 / Serving Size: 1/4 recipe**

# broiled sole with red pepper coulis

**4** red bell peppers
**1 lb** sole fillets
**1 tsp** extra virgin olive oil
**1 large clove** garlic, minced
**1/4 tsp** fine sea salt
**1/8 tsp** freshly ground black pepper

1. Place whole peppers directly on a grill, gas burner, or under your broiler. Roast until they are completely blackened on the outside. Place in a bowl and cover tightly with plastic wrap for at least 15 minutes. Once cooled, you can peel away the blackened skin.

2. Place the roasted pepper in the food processor and puree until fine.

3. Mix the extra virgin olive oil with the garlic, salt, and pepper. Spread on one side of fish and broil until golden. Serve with pureed roasted red peppers.

## Cook's Tip

*Why not roast extra peppers and keep them in your fridge or freezer to jazz up other dishes?*

**Exchanges/Choices: 2 Vegetable, 3 Lean Meat**
**Calories 155, Calories from Fat 25,**
**Total Fat 3 g, Saturated Fat 0.6 g, Trans Fat 0 g,**
**Cholesterol 60 mg, Sodium 245 mg, Total Carbohydrate 9 g,**
**Dietary Fiber 3 g, Sugars 6 g, Protein 23 g**

*The flavors of the fennel, figs, & blood orange combine perfectly to create this lovely **Fish Fillet with Fennel, Figs & Orange**.*

**Serves 4 / Serving Size: 1/4 recipe**
# fish fillet with fennel, figs & orange

- **1 Tbsp** extra virgin olive oil
- **1 cup** chopped onion (about 1 medium)
- **1 cup** chopped fennel
- **1/2 cup** chicken or fish stock
- **1/2 cup** dry white wine
- **2 oz** chopped dried figs
- **1 lb** thin white fish fillets (flounder or sole)
- **2** blood oranges, 1 juiced and 1 cut in half and sliced (navel oranges will also work)

1. Place olive oil in sauté pan. Add onion and cook until onion begins to turn brown on the edges. Add fennel and cook 2–3 minutes or until fennel and onion are tender.

2. Add stock, wine, and figs. Bring to a boil.

3. Place fish on top of this mixture. Cover and steam until fish flakes with a fork, approximately 3–5 minutes depending on thickness of fish.

4. Serve fish over the fennel and fig relish. Drizzle with juice of 1 orange and garnish each serving with remaining orange slices.

EXCHANGES/CHOICES:  1 FRUIT, 1 VEGETABLE, 3 LEAN MEAT
CALORIES 225,  CALORIES FROM FAT 45,
TOTAL FAT 5 G,  SATURATED FAT 0.8 G,  TRANS FAT 0 G,
CHOLESTEROL 60 MG,  SODIUM 230 MG,  TOTAL CARBOHYDRATE 20 G,
DIETARY FIBER 3 G,  SUGARS 14 G,  PROTEIN 23 G

*"Francaise" is a must in any cook's repertoire because it is so easy and so quick. This* **Flounder Francaise** *recipe is no exception.*

**Serves 4 / Serving Size: 1/4 recipe**

# flounder francaise

**1 Tbsp** extra virgin olive oil

**1 Tbsp** canola oil

**1/4 cup** Wondra flour (all-purpose will work also)

**1/4 tsp** fine sea salt

**1/4 tsp** freshly ground black pepper

**2** egg whites

**1 lb** flounder fillets (4 pieces)

**1/2 cup** dry white wine (Pinot Grigio or Sauvignon Blanc)

**2** lemons, juiced

**1 Tbsp** minced fresh Italian parsley

**1 Tbsp** capers (optional)

1. Place olive oil and canola oil in large nonstick sauté pan. Heat until oil has a slight sizzle.

2. Place flour, salt, and pepper in one dish. Place egg whites in second dish. Dip fish in flour and then egg. Place fish in hot pan and brown on first side, approximately 3 minutes. Turn and brown on second side.

3. Add wine and lemon juice. Cook 1–2 minutes to reduce slightly. Sprinkle with parsley. If using capers, add with wine and lemon juice. Serve immediately so that the egg crust does not get soggy.

## Cook's Tip

*You want to cook with a wine that is good enough to drink, not cooking wine, which is cheap wine loaded with salt.*

EXCHANGES/CHOICES: 1/2 CARBOHYDRATE, 3 LEAN MEAT, 1 FAT
CALORIES 210, CALORIES FROM FAT 70,
TOTAL FAT 8 G, SATURATED FAT 1 G, TRANS FAT 0 G,
CHOLESTEROL 60 MG, SODIUM 275 MG, TOTAL CARBOHYDRATE 8 G,
DIETARY FIBER 0 G, SUGARS 1 G, PROTEIN 24 G

*This Flounder Spinach Rolls with a Shallot White Wine Sauce*
*dish has a variety of wonderful flavors that combine for a beautiful end result.*

**Serves 4 / Serving Size: 1/4 recipe**

# flounder spinach rolls
## with a shallot white wine sauce

**1 lb** flounder fillets, preferably 4 pieces

**1/4 tsp** fine sea salt

**1/8 tsp** freshly ground pepper

**1 (5 oz) bag** baby spinach

**2 Tbsp** grated Parmigiano-Reggiano

**1 cup** dry white wine (Orvieto or Pinot Grigio)

**1/2 cup** chicken or vegetable stock

**1** shallot, minced

**1/2 cup** roasted soy nuts, crushed

1. Preheat over to 350°.

2. Lay fish fillets out on work surface. Season lightly with salt and pepper. Lay several spinach leaves on top of each fillet. Sprinkle equally with Parmigiano-Reggiano. Roll each fillet and secure with toothpick.

3. Place remaining spinach in the bottom of the baking dish. Top with fish and pour the white wine and stock around. Sprinkle with minced shallot. Cover and bake 30 minutes. Sprinkle with soy nuts before serving.

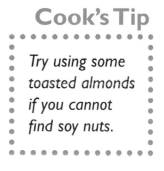

## Cook's Tip

*Try using some toasted almonds if you cannot find soy nuts.*

**EXCHANGES/CHOICES:** 1/2 CARBOHYDRATE, 4 LEAN MEAT
**CALORIES** 235, **CALORIES FROM FAT** 45,
**TOTAL FAT** 5 G, **SATURATED FAT** 1.4 G, **TRANS FAT** 0 G,
**CHOLESTEROL** 60 MG, **SODIUM** 530 MG, **TOTAL CARBOHYDRATE** 10 G,
**DIETARY FIBER** 5 G, **SUGARS** 3 G, **PROTEIN** 33 G

*This **Flounder Stuffed with Couscous** dish has many of my favorite flavors and is also lovely to look at. The mango and pomegranate are like little jewels against the couscous.*

**Serves 4 / Serving Size: 1/4 recipe**

# flounder stuffed with couscous

**1 cup** uncooked whole-wheat couscous

**1/2 cup** pomegranate seeds

**1/2 cup** diced mango (can be purchased in the refrigerated produce section, if fresh is not available)

**1/4 cup** fresh mint leaves

**1/4 cup** rice wine vinegar

**1/4 tsp** fine sea salt

**1/8 tsp** freshly ground black pepper

**1 lb** flounder fillets

**1/2 cup** dry white wine or fish or chicken stock

1. Preheat oven to 375°.

2. Bring 2 cups of water to a boil. Add couscous. Stir well. Set aside and let stand approximately 3 minutes until all liquid is evaporated. Add pomegranate seeds, mango, mint, and vinegar. Mix well. Season with salt and pepper.

3. Lay fish fillets on flat surface. Top each fillet with the couscous and roll up. Secure with toothpicks. Place in baking dish in single layer. Pour wine around fish. Cover with aluminum foil and bake for 20 minutes.

4. Serve fish with remaining couscous and pomegranate seeds. Garnish with additional mint leaves.

**Cook's Tip**

*If you can't find mangos in your grocery store, a peach is an excellent mango substitute.*

EXCHANGES/CHOICES: 2 STARCH, 1/2 FRUIT, 3 LEAN MEAT
CALORIES 280, CALORIES FROM FAT 25,
TOTAL FAT 3 G, SATURATED FAT 0.6 G, TRANS FAT 0 G,
CHOLESTEROL 60 MG, SODIUM 250 MG, TOTAL CARBOHYDRATE 36 G,
DIETARY FIBER 4 G, SUGARS 7 G, PROTEIN 27 G

Garlic Shrimp on a Cucumber Flower, page 3

Scallop Seviche Martini,
page 10

Grilled Tuna Over Baby Greens, page 26

Warm Shrimp and Bean
Salad, page 36

Salmon with Black Bean Salsa, page 54

Bloody Mary Shrimp,
page 115

Risotto with Shrimp and Lemon, page 122

Lemon Yogurt Pound Cake, page 150

*Try these* **Oven-Baked Herb-Crusted Fish Fillets** *instead of a fried dish. They are healthier and very delicious.*

**Serves 4 / Serving Size: 1/4 recipe**

# oven-baked herb-crusted fish fillets

**1/2 cup** pignoli (pine nuts)
**1 cup** fresh bread crumbs
**2 Tbsp** freshly grated Parmigiano-Reggiano
**1/4 tsp** fine sea salt
**1/8 tsp** freshly ground pepper
**4** egg whites
**1 lb** fish fillet of your choice (flounder, sole, tilapia)

1. Preheat oven to 425°.

2. Line a baking sheet with parchment paper or foil.

3. Place pignoli in a plastic bag and crush with a meat mallet or rolling pin. Mix bread crumbs, Parmigiano-Reggiano, pignoli, salt, and pepper together in a pie plate.

4. Place egg whites in another pie plate. Dip fish in egg whites.

5. Dip fish in bread crumbs and place on parchment paper or foil. Bake for 20 minutes or until fish flakes with fork and crust is golden.

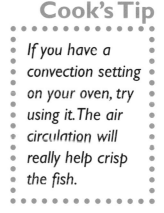

## Cook's Tip

*If you have a convection setting on your oven, try using it. The air circulation will really help crisp the fish.*

EXCHANGES/CHOICES: 1/2 STARCH, 4 LEAN MEAT, 1/2 FAT
CALORIES 230, CALORIES FROM FAT 100,
TOTAL FAT 11 G, SATURATED FAT 1.2 G, TRANS FAT 0 G,
CHOLESTEROL 60 MG, SODIUM 305 MG, TOTAL CARBOHYDRATE 6 G,
DIETARY FIBER 1 G, SUGARS 1 G, PROTEIN 27 G

*Whole grains are important in our diet and crunch is important for texture*
*— this **Oven-Fried Catfish with Tortilla Chips** combines both.*

**Serves 4 / Serving Size: 1/4 recipe**

# oven-fried catfish with tortilla chips

**2 cups** multi-grain tortilla chips (about 1 1/4 ounce)
**1/4 tsp** fine sea salt
**1/4 tsp** freshly ground pepper
**2 tsp** Mexican seasoning
**2** egg whites
**1 lb** catfish fillet
Salsa (optional for serving)

1. Preheat oven to 400°.

2. Place tortilla chips in food processor fitted with steel blade and finely chop to 1/2 cup. Add salt, pepper, and Mexican seasoning. Place in shallow dish or pie plate.

3. Place egg whites in shallow dish or pie plate.

4. Dip fish fillets in egg and then crumb mixture. Place on parchment-lined baking sheet and bake at 400° for 15 minutes, until crispy. Serve with your favorite salsa.

## Cook's Tip

*Any nonfat, fresh salsa will work, or simply chop some tomatoes, cilantro, and onion and add a splash of lime juice.*

**EXCHANGES/CHOICES:** 1/2 STARCH, 3 LEAN MEAT, 1 FAT
**CALORIES** 210, **CALORIES FROM FAT** 100,
**TOTAL FAT** 11 G, **SATURATED FAT** 2.1 G, **TRANS FAT** 0 G,
**CHOLESTEROL** 65 MG, **SODIUM** 300 MG, **TOTAL CARBOHYDRATE** 6 G,
**DIETARY FIBER** 1 G, **SUGARS** 0 G, **PROTEIN** 21 G

*Nuts are a wonderful pantry ingredient that really dress up this simple **Pecan-Crusted Orange Roughy** recipe.*

**Serves 4 / Serving Size: 1/4 recipe**

# pecan-crusted orange roughy

Cooking spray
**1 lb** orange roughy fillet (or lemon sole or flounder)
**1/2 cup** crushed pecans
**1/2 cup** orange juice

1. Preheat oven to 375°.

2. Spray baking dish lightly with cooking spray.

3. Lay fish fillet in baking dish in single layer. Top with crushed pecans. Pour orange juice around fish.

4. Bake for about 15 minutes.

## Cook's Tip

*Any white fillet can be substituted for the orange roughy in this recipe.*

EXCHANGES/CHOICES: 1/2 CARBOHYDRATE, 3 LEAN MEAT, 1 FAT
CALORIES 205, CALORIES FROM FAT 100,
TOTAL FAT 11 G, SATURATED FAT 0.9 G, TRANS FAT 0 G,
CHOLESTEROL 70 MG, SODIUM 60 MG, TOTAL CARBOHYDRATE 5 G,
DIETARY FIBER 1 G, SUGARS 4 G, PROTEIN 22 G

*There are some things that you just can't live without and good prosciutto is one of them! This **Prosciutto-Wrapped Tilapia** is great because it combines prosciutto with the delightful taste of tilapia and arugula.*

**Serves 4 / Serving Size: 1/4 recipe**

# prosciutto-wrapped tilapia

**4 oz** imported Italian prosciutto, thinly sliced
**1 lb** tilapia fillets, cut in half lengthwise (about 2 large fillets)
**4 cups** fresh arugula (about 2 bunches)
**1 cup** white wine
**1** lemon, juiced
**1/4 tsp** freshly ground black pepper

1. Divide prosciutto into 4 servings. Lay prosciutto out on work surface. Top with a piece of fish. Top with enough arugula to cover fish. Wrap prosciutto around fish and arugula.

2. Preheat nonstick sauté pan. Add fish bundles and brown on bottom. Once they are nicely browned on bottom, add white wine and cover. Cook on medium heat for 5–8 minutes, depending on the thickness of the fish.

3. Remove fish to plate. Reduce remaining wine sauce if desired. Serve with remaining arugula, tossed with the lemon juice and pepper.

## Cook's Tip

*Chicken stock or dry white vermouth can be substituted for white wine if you don't have any in your pantry.*

**EXCHANGES/CHOICES: 4 LEAN MEAT**
**CALORIES** 200, **CALORIES FROM FAT** 55,
**TOTAL FAT** 6 G, **SATURATED FAT** 2 G, **TRANS FAT** 0 G,
**CHOLESTEROL** 90 MG, **SODIUM** 545 MG, **TOTAL CARBOHYDRATE** 3 G,
**DIETARY FIBER** 1 G, **SUGARS** 1 G, **PROTEIN** 31 G

*Pesto originated in Genoa, Italy, and is a lifesaver in the kitchen.  It gives*

*a lift to just about anything, and this* **Sole Genovese** *is no exception.*

**Serves 4 / Serving Size: 1/4 recipe**

# sole genovese

**1 lb** sole fillets (dover, lemon, grey)

**2 oz** Pesto (recipe on page **142**) or prepare your own

**8 oz** fresh tomatoes (heirloom tomatoes are a nice choice)

1. Lay sole out on large platter and coat evenly with Pesto (recipe on page 142).

2. Preheat sauté pan. Add fish and cook until the Pesto begins to brown. Turn and cook second side until fish flakes with fork, about 3 minutes on each side.  Serve with sliced tomatoes.

## Cook's Tip

*There is nothing like preparing your own pesto, except maybe making double, since it freezes so well.*

EXCHANGES/CHOICES:  3 LEAN MEAT, 1/2 FAT
CALORIES 170,  CALORIES FROM FAT 65,
TOTAL FAT 7 G,  SATURATED FAT 1.2 G,  TRANS FAT 0 G,
CHOLESTEROL 60 MG,  SODIUM 105 MG,  TOTAL CARBOHYDRATE 3 G,
DIETARY FIBER 1 G,  SUGARS 1 G,  PROTEIN 23 G

*Some food combinations are perfect, and the tomato and basil in this* **Sole with Cherry Tomato & Basil** *are at the top of the list.*

**Serves 4 / Serving Size: 1/4 recipe**

# sole with cherry tomato & basil

**1 oz** uncooked polenta or cornmeal

**1/4 tsp** fine sea salt

**1/8 tsp** freshly ground black pepper

**1 lb** sole fillets (dover, lemon, grey)

**1 Tbsp** extra virgin olive oil

**1 large clove** garlic, peeled and crushed

**1 cup** chopped fresh basil

**1 cup** sliced cherry tomatoes

**2 oz** dry white wine

1. Place cornmeal in shallow dish or pie pan. Add salt and pepper. Dip both sides of fish in cornmeal.

2. Place olive oil in sauté pan. Heat and add fish. Brown fish on one side and turn over. While browning on other side, add crushed garlic, basil, and tomatoes to pan surface so that they cook alongside the fish.

3. Cook until fish flakes with fork, about 3 minutes on each side. Add white wine and heat thoroughly.

4. Serve with whole grain pasta, if desired.

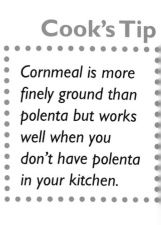

**Cook's Tip**

*Cornmeal is more finely ground than polenta but works well when you don't have polenta in your kitchen.*

**EXCHANGES/CHOICES:** 1/2 STARCH, 3 LEAN MEAT
**CALORIES** 175, **CALORIES FROM FAT** 45,
**TOTAL FAT** 5 G, **SATURATED FAT** 0.8 G, **TRANS FAT** 0 G,
**CHOLESTEROL** 60 MG, **SODIUM** 245 MG, **TOTAL CARBOHYDRATE** 8 G,
**DIETARY FIBER** 1 G, **SUGARS** 1 G, **PROTEIN** 23 G

*Color not only enhances our plate visually, but the bright colors in this dish add to the nutritional profile of this* **Tilapia Balsamico** *recipe.*

**Serves 4 / Serving Size: 1/4 recipe**

# tilapia balsamico

**1/2 cup** balsamic vinegar

**1 lb** tilapia fillet

**1/2 tsp** fine sea salt

**1/4 tsp** freshly ground pepper

**1 Tbsp** extra virgin olive oil

**2** shallots, minced

**1 clove** garlic, minced

**4** small zucchini, 4–6 inches long, sliced into 1/4-inch rounds

**3/4 cup** dry white wine (Pinot Grigio or Sauvignon Blanc)

**1 (7 oz) jar** roasted peppers

**1/2 cup** fresh basil, chopped or chiffonade

1. Place vinegar in small saucepan and cook for 15–20 minutes, until reduced to 1/4 cup or the vinegar coats the back of a spoon.

2. Season fish with salt and pepper and place in refrigerator.

3. Place oil, shallot, and garlic in sauté pan. Cook until shallot becomes translucent. Add zucchini and sauté 1–2 minutes. Remove from pan.

4. Add fish and sauté until golden on each side. Add white wine to deglaze pan. Add zucchini, roasted peppers, and fresh basil. Heat thoroughly. Remove to plate and drizzle with balsamic reduction.

5. Serve with whole-wheat pasta, rice, couscous, or Italian bread.

EXCHANGES/CHOICES: 1/2 CARBOHYDRATE, 2 VEGETABLE, 3 LEAN MEAT
CALORIES 225, CALORIES FROM FAT 55,
TOTAL FAT 6 G, SATURATED FAT 1.5 G, TRANS FAT 0 G,
CHOLESTEROL 75 MG, SODIUM 440 MG, TOTAL CARBOHYDRATE 16 G,
DIETARY FIBER 2 G, SUGARS 8 G, PROTEIN 25 G

*Cream sauce can be enjoyed when made with "lighter" ingredients, just like it has been in this delightful recipe for **Tilapia with Artichokes and Peas In a Light Herb Cream Sauce**.*

**Serves 4 / Serving Size: 1/4 recipe**

# tilapia with artichokes and peas in a light herb cream sauce

**1/2 cup** Wondra flour

**1/4 tsp** fine sea salt

**1 lb** tilapia fillet

**1/8 tsp** freshly ground pepper

**1 tsp** extra virgin olive oil

**4 cloves** garlic, minced

**1/2 cup** fresh basil, chopped

**1/2 cup** Italian parsley, chopped

**1** shallot, minced

**10 oz** frozen artichoke hearts, defrosted enough to break apart

**10 oz** petite peas

**1/2 cup** chicken stock

**12 oz** evaporated skim milk

1. Place flour in shallow dish. Add salt and pepper. Dip fish fillets in flour.

2. Heat sauté pan and add olive oil. Add fish fillets and cook until golden on first side. Turn fish and add garlic to pan surface so it cooks while the fish is cooking on the second side.

3. Add basil, parsley, shallot, artichokes, peas, stock, and evaporated skim milk. Cook on low to medium (just below boil) for 10 minutes.

4. Serve over couscous, rice, pasta, or polenta.

## Cook's Tip

*I like to keep evaporated skim milk in the pantry for emergencies when there is no milk on hand.*

**EXCHANGES/CHOICES: 1 STARCH, 1 FAT-FREE MILK, 1 VEGETABLE, 3 LEAN MEAT**
**CALORIES 325, CALORIES FROM FAT 40,**
**TOTAL FAT 4.5 G, SATURATED FAT 1.3 G, TRANS FAT 0 G,**
**CHOLESTEROL 80 MG, SODIUM 470 MG, TOTAL CARBOHYDRATE 37 G,**
**DIETARY FIBER 7 G, SUGARS 16 G, PROTEIN 37 G**

*I invited friends over to "taste" this* **Tilapia with Shiitake & Rosemary** *for me and they insisted that it had to be in this book.*

**Serves 4 / Serving Size: 1/4 recipe**

# tilapia with shiitake & rosemary

**1 lb** tilapia fillet
**1/4 tsp** fine sea salt
**1/8 tsp** freshly ground pepper
**1 Tbsp** extra virgin olive oil
**1 clove** garlic, crushed and peeled
**1 cup** sliced shiitake mushrooms
**1 cup** fresh basil
**2 Tbsp** fresh rosemary leaves
**1 cup** dry white wine (not Chardonnay)
**1 cup** fish, chicken, or vegetable stock
**1/2 cup** chopped sun-dried tomatoes (not in oil)
**2 Tbsp** grated Parmigiano-Reggiano (optional)

1. Lay fillets out on work surface. Season lightly with salt and pepper.

2. Place olive oil in pan. Add garlic and mushrooms and cook about 1 minute until garlic becomes fragrant but not brown. Add basil and rosemary and sauté 1 minute. Push this mixture to the side.

3. Add fish and cook on first side. Turn fish and add wine, stock, and sun-dried tomatoes. Cook until fish flakes with a fork, approximately 5 minutes. Garnish with grated Parmigiano-Reggiano.

4. Serve with crusty multi-grain bread, multi-grain small pasta, or whole-wheat couscous.

EXCHANGES/CHOICES: 2 VEGETABLE, 3 LEAN MEAT
CALORIES 205, CALORIES FROM FAT 55,
TOTAL FAT 6 G, SATURATED FAT 1.5 G, TRANS FAT 0 G,
CHOLESTEROL 75 MG, SODIUM 185 MG, TOTAL CARBOHYDRATE 9 G,
DIETARY FIBER 2 G, SUGARS 3 G, PROTEIN 24 G

# Chapter 6:

# THICK FILLETS

*The shiitake mushrooms and snow peas in this **Asian-Style Skillet** are a nice change of pace from more commonly consumed veggies.*

**Serves 4 / Serving Size: 1/4 recipe**

# asian-style skillet

**2 tsp** canola oil (divided use)

**4 tsp** szechwan seasoning blend

**1 lb** thick fillet (cod, snapper, thick flounder, or tilapia)

**4 oz** snow peas

**4 oz** shiitake mushrooms

**1 cup** dry white wine or stock

**1 1/2 cups** chopped tomato (about 1 medium)

1. Rub 1 tsp canola oil and seasoning blend over fillet.

2. Cut snow peas in half lengthwise. Slice shiitake mushrooms into 1/2-inch pieces.

3. Place 1 tsp canola oil in large skillet. Heat and add fish. Brown first side of fish and turn. While second side is browning, add snow peas and shiitake mushrooms. Cook 2–3 minutes and add wine and tomatoes. Continue to cook until fish flakes with a fork.

4. Serve with Mushroom Garlic-Scented Rice (recipe on page 153).

## Cook's Tip

*You can easily substitute cremini mushrooms for shiitake if necessary.*

EXCHANGES/CHOICES: 2 VEGETABLE, 3 LEAN MEAT
CALORIES 170, CALORIES FROM FAT 30,
TOTAL FAT 3.5 G, SATURATED FAT 0.4 G, TRANS FAT 0 G,
CHOLESTEROL 50 MG, SODIUM 75 MG, TOTAL CARBOHYDRATE 8 G,
DIETARY FIBER 2 G, SUGARS 4 G, PROTEIN 22 G

*Inspired by an Italian recipe, this **Baked FIllet with Bread Crumbs** dish is delicious, quick, and easy-to-make.*

**Serves 4 / Serving Size: 1/4 recipe**

# baked fillet with bread crumbs

Cooking spray

**1 lb** thick fillet, cut into 4 servings (cod, snapper, thick flounder, or thick tilapia)

**1/2 cup** whole-grain bread crumbs

**1/4 cup** fresh Italian parsley leaves

**1 Tbsp** fresh marjoram or oregano leaves

**1/4 cup** fresh basil leaves

**1 large clove** garlic, crushed and peeled

1. Preheat oven to 400°.

2. Spray baking dish lightly with cooking spray.

3. Place bread crumbs, parsley, marjoram, basil, and garlic in food processor and pulse until the herbs are incorporated into the bread crumbs.

4. Dip fish into bread crumb and herb mixture. Place in prepared baking dish and place in preheated oven. Bake 15 minutes.

5. Serve on top of a mixed green salad with Basic Vinaigrette (recipe on page 138).

EXCHANGES/CHOICES: 1/2 STARCH, 3 LEAN MEAT
CALORIES 170, CALORIES FROM FAT 25,
TOTAL FAT 3 G, SATURATED FAT 0.4 G, TRANS FAT 0 G,
CHOLESTEROL 35 MG, SODIUM 75 MG, TOTAL CARBOHYDRATE 9 G,
DIETARY FIBER 2 G, SUGARS 1 G, PROTEIN 25 G

*By lightening up usually high-fat coconut milk with chicken or fish stock, you can preserve its wonderful taste while making this* **Coconut Stir-Fry with Orange Roughy** *both delicious and healthy.*

**Serves 4 / Serving Size: 1/4 recipe**

# coconut stir-fry with orange roughy

**1/3 cup** light coconut milk
**2 tsp** green curry paste
**1 cup** chicken or fish stock
**1 tsp** canola oil
**3 cups** sliced red bell pepper
**2 cups** snow peas, julienned
**1 clove** garlic, crushed
**1 lb** orange roughy fillet

1. Combine coconut milk, curry paste, and chicken stock. Mix well and set aside.

2. Place canola oil in sauté pan. Heat and add bell pepper, snow peas, and garlic. Stir-fry about 3 minutes, until vegetables begin to soften. Add fish and cook until lightly browned. Push fish and vegetables to the side.

3. Add coconut milk, curry, and chicken stock. Turn heat to high and bring sauce to boil. Heat thoroughly and stir into fish and vegetables.

4. Serve with jasmine rice.

## Cook's Tip

*Jasmine rice is a wonderful scented, sweet rice that is very versatile.*

EXCHANGES/CHOICES: 2 VEGETABLE, 3 LEAN MEAT
CALORIES 175, CALORIES FROM FAT 30,
TOTAL FAT 3.5 G, SATURATED FAT 0.8 G, TRANS FAT 0 G,
CHOLESTEROL 70 MG, SODIUM 400 MG, TOTAL CARBOHYDRATE 11 G,
DIETARY FIBER 4 G, SUGARS 7 G, PROTEIN 24 G

*Incorporating more dark leafy vegetables into your diet is easy with this **Cod with Pasta and Mixed Greens** recipe.*

**Serves 4 / Serving Size: 1/4 recipe**

# cod with pasta and mixed greens

1 small bunch arugula, chopped (about 1 cup)

1 (6 oz) bag baby spinach

1 small bunch watercress, chopped (about 1 cup)

1 lb thick fillet of cod

1/4 tsp fine sea salt

1/4 tsp freshly ground pepper

1/2 lb penne pasta

1 cup nonfat cottage cheese

2 oz light cream cheese

1 (12 oz) can evaporated skim milk

1/2 cup coarsely grated asiago cheese

1/2 Tbsp extra virgin olive oil

2 cloves garlic, minced

1/2 cup chicken or vegetable stock

1. Wash and coarsely chop greens. Dry them well (a salad spinner helps). Cut cod into bite-sized pieces. Season with salt and pepper. Set aside.

2. Set a large pot of water to boil on the stove. When the water boils, add pasta and cook to al dente stage.

3. In the meantime, place cottage cheese in food processor and process until smooth. Add cream cheese in 1-inch cubes and process until smooth. Add skim milk and asiago cheese. Mix thoroughly. Set aside.

4. Thinly cover bottom of sauté pan with olive oil. Sauté cod and garlic until garlic becomes fragrant, about 2 minutes. Add stock to deglaze pan. Add greens, cover, and steam about 2 minutes until wilted.

5. Toss with pasta and cheese sauce and serve immediately.

EXCHANGES/CHOICES: 3 STARCH, 1 FAT-FREE MILK, 4 LEAN MEAT
CALORIES 520, CALORIES FROM FAT 80,
TOTAL FAT 9 G, SATURATED FAT 4.3 G, TRANS FAT 0 G,
CHOLESTEROL 75 MG, SODIUM 850 MG, TOTAL CARBOHYDRATE 60 G,
DIETARY FIBER 3 G, SUGARS 15 G, PROTEIN 47 G

*Primavera means springtime. This quick **Fillet Primavera** reflects the flavors of spring, but you can vary the vegetables by using whatever you like, such as green beans, carrots, broccoli, and much more.*

**Serves 4 / Serving Size: 1/4 recipe**

# fillet primavera

**1/2 cup** Wondra flour
**1/2 tsp** fine sea salt
**1/4 tsp** freshly ground pepper
**1 lb** thick white fillet (cod, halibut, or large tilapia)
**1 Tbsp** extra virgin olive oil
**2 cloves** garlic, minced
**1 cup** petite frozen peas, uncooked

**1 (10 oz) box** frozen artichoke hearts, uncooked
**1 lb** thin asparagus, cut into thirds
**1/2 cup** fish or chicken stock
**1/2 cup** white wine
**1/4 cup** flat Italian parsley, roughly chopped
**1/4 cup** chopped fresh basil

1. Mix flour, salt, and pepper in shallow bowl. Dip fish in flour and coat both sides.

2. Place olive oil in sauté pan and heat to medium. Add fish and cook until golden on first side. Turn. While fish is browning on second side, add garlic to pan surface. When garlic becomes fragrant, add peas, artichokes, asparagus, stock, and wine. Cover and cook 3–5 minutes until asparagus is tender and fish is cooked through and flakes with a fork.

3. Sprinkle with parsley and basil and serve over small pasta, rice, or couscous.

## Cook's Tip

*Wondra, commonly known as instant flour, is a very fine granular flour that is also used to make smooth sauces. This type of flour will absorb less oil in the preparation process.*

**EXCHANGES/CHOICES: 1 STARCH, 1 VEGETABLE, 3 LEAN MEAT**
**CALORIES 245, CALORIES FROM FAT 45,**
**TOTAL FAT 5 G, SATURATED FAT 0.6 G, TRANS FAT 0 G,**
**CHOLESTEROL 50 MG, SODIUM 365 MG, TOTAL CARBOHYDRATE 23 G,**
**DIETARY FIBER 6 G, SUGARS 4 G, PROTEIN 27 G**

*Prosecco is a light, dry Italian sparkling wine from the Veneto. Not only lower in alcohol, it is priced affordably so you can make this* **Fillet with Prosecco & Mushrooms** *as often as you want.*

**Serves 4 / Serving Size: 1/4 recipe**

# fillet with prosecco & mushrooms

**10 oz** cremini or white button mushrooms

**2 cloves** garlic, minced

**1 oz** Parmigiano-Reggiano

**1 Tbsp** extra virgin olive oil

**1 lb** thick white fillet, cut into 4 portions (cod, snapper, thick flounder, or thick tilapia)

**1 cup** sliced cherry tomatoes, about 1/2 pint

**1 cup** Prosecco wine

1. Place mushrooms, garlic, and Parmigiano-Reggiano in food processor fitted with steel blade. Process to a fine paste.

2. Heat olive oil in large nonstick sauté pan. Add fish and brown 2–3 minutes on first side. Turn fish and brown on second side. While fish is cooking, place mushroom paste and tomatoes around fish in pan. Add wine and bring to a boil. Reduce heat to low. Simmer 5 minutes to cook mushrooms and tomatoes.

3. Serve over whole-grain pasta, if desired.

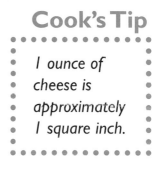

**Cook's Tip**

*1 ounce of cheese is approximately 1 square inch.*

**EXCHANGES/CHOICES: 1 VEGETABLE, 3 LEAN MEAT, 1/2 FAT**
**CALORIES 195, CALORIES FROM FAT 55,**
**TOTAL FAT 6 G, SATURATED FAT 1.7 G, TRANS FAT 0 G,**
**CHOLESTEROL 55 MG, SODIUM 130 MG, TOTAL CARBOHYDRATE 5 G,**
**DIETARY FIBER 1 G, SUGARS 2 G, PROTEIN 25 G**

*When you cook with a lot of color, you automatically increase the variety of nutrients in your diet. This **Fillet with Shallot, Zucchini & Tomato** dish is filled with color and nutrition.*

**Serves 4 / Serving Size: 1/4 recipe**

# fillet with shallot, zucchini & tomato

**1 lb** thick white fillet of fish, cut into 4 portions (cod, snapper, thick flounder, or thick tilapia)

**3/4 tsp** fine sea salt

**1/4 tsp** freshly ground pepper

**1 tsp** extra virgin olive oil

**2** shallots, minced

**1 clove** garlic, minced

**4** small zucchini, 4–6 inches long, sliced into 1/4-inch rounds

**3/4 cup** dry white wine or chicken or fish stock

**4** very ripe plum tomatoes, chopped

**1/2 cup** fresh basil, chopped

1. Season each piece of fish with salt and pepper and refrigerate.

2. Heat sauté pan and lightly film with olive oil. Sauté shallot and garlic until shallot starts to become translucent. Add zucchini and sauté 1–2 minutes. Remove from pan.

3. Add fish and sauté until golden on each side. Add white wine or stock to deglaze pan. Add chopped tomatoes and fresh basil. Heat thoroughly.

4. Serve with a pasta, rice, couscous, or crusty whole-grain Italian bread.

EXCHANGES/CHOICES: 2 VEGETABLE, 3 LEAN MEAT
CALORIES 195, CALORIES FROM FAT 40,
TOTAL FAT 4.5 G, SATURATED FAT 0.7 G, TRANS FAT 0 G,
CHOLESTEROL 35 MG, SODIUM 520 MG, TOTAL CARBOHYDRATE 10 G,
DIETARY FIBER 3 G, SUGARS 4 G, PROTEIN 26 G

*The tomatillos in this **Fillet with Tomatillo Salsa** give a snap of flavor that is well complimented by the tomatoes, garlic, lime, and cilantro.*

**Serves 4 / Serving Size: 1/4 recipe**

# fillet with tomatillo salsa

**1 lb** thick white fillet, cut into 4 portions (cod, snapper, thick flounder, or thick tilapia)

**1/2 tsp** ground cumin

**1 tsp** canola oil

**3 cups** chopped fresh tomatillos (about 1 lb)

**2 cloves** garlic, minced

**1 cup** chopped grape tomatoes (about 1/2 pint)

**1/4 cup** fresh lime juice

**1 cup** fresh cilantro leaves, roughly chopped

1. Sprinkle fillet with cumin. Set aside.

2. Place canola oil in nonstick sauté pan and heat over medium heat. Add tomatillos and garlic. Sauté 3–4 minutes until tomatillos begin to soften. Add tomatoes, lime juice, and cilantro. Sauté 2 minutes and mix well. Push this mixture to the side of the pan.

3. Add fish and sauté about 3–4 minutes on first side. Turn and brown on second side. While fish is browning, spread sauce around fish.

4. Place a portion of fish on each dinner plate and top with sauce. Serve with polenta or rice. Garnish with additional cilantro, slices of lime, and a light sprinkling of grated low-fat cheddar cheese.

## Cook's Tip

*Fresh tomatillos can be found in the fresh produce section of most grocery stores.*

**EXCHANGES/CHOICES: 2 VEGETABLE, 3 LEAN MEAT**
**CALORIES 180, CALORIES FROM FAT 45,**
**TOTAL FAT 5 G, SATURATED FAT 0.6 G, TRANS FAT 0 G,**
**CHOLESTEROL 35 MG, SODIUM 70 MG, TOTAL CARBOHYDRATE 9 G,**
**DIETARY FIBER 3 G, SUGARS 6 G, PROTEIN 25 G**

*The radicchio in this **Fish A La Mediterraneo** recipe is a beautiful deep red color when fresh and uncooked, but when it is cooked, the color changes to a savory brown and the flavor becomes sweeter.*

**Serves 4 / Serving Size: 1/4 recipe**

# fish a la mediterraneo

**1 Tbsp** extra virgin olive oil

**2 cloves** garlic, crushed and chopped

**2 cups** thinly sliced fennel (about 1 small or medium bulb)

**1 lb** thick white fillet of fish, cut into 4 portions (cod, snapper, thick flounder, or tilapia)

**1/4 tsp** fine sea salt

**1/2 tsp** freshly ground black pepper

**1/4 cup** fresh basil, chopped

**2 cups** thinly sliced radicchio (1 small head)

**1/2 cup** white wine

**1/4 cup** orange juice

**1** navel orange, sliced

1. Heat olive oil, garlic, and fennel in large sauté pan. Cook about 5 minutes until fennel begins to brown on the edges. Push to the side of the pan and add fish.

2. Cook fish until first side is golden. Turn. While fish is browning on second side, sprinkle with salt and pepper and add basil, radicchio, wine, and orange juice. Toss well and cook until radicchio is slightly wilted and the color begins to change from red to brown.

3. Divide the fish and vegetable mixture among 4 dinner plates and top with orange sections.

## Cook's Tip

*A navel orange is recommended because it is seedless but any orange will do, if seeds are removed.*

**EXCHANGES/CHOICES: 1/2 FRUIT, 1 VEGETABLE, 3 LEAN MEAT**
**CALORIES 180, CALORIES FROM FAT 40,**
**TOTAL FAT 4.5 G, SATURATED FAT 0.6 G, TRANS FAT 0 G,**
**CHOLESTEROL 50 MG, SODIUM 245 MG, TOTAL CARBOHYDRATE 11 G,**
**DIETARY FIBER 3 G, SUGARS 7 G, PROTEIN 22 G**

*A piquant marinade combined with a simple cooking method creates a complex taste sensation in this **Grilled Sea Bass with Vegetables**.*

**Serves 4 / Serving Size: 1/4 recipe**

# grilled sea bass with vegetables

**piquant marinade**

- **2 Tbsp** capers
- **2 Tbsp** olive oil
- **2 Tbsp** black olive paste or 1/3 cup finely chopped black olives
- **2 Tbsp** balsamic vinegar
- **2 Tbsp** fresh lemon juice
- **1/2 cup** fresh oregano

- **1 lb** Chilean sea bass
- **1** fennel bulb, sliced 1/4-inch thick
- **1** small eggplant, sliced 1/4-inch thick
- **1** small zucchini, sliced 1/2-inch thick lengthwise
- **2** red bell peppers, cored, seeded, and sliced into 1/4-inch rounds
- **1** large onion, sliced 1/4-inch thick
- **2** lemons, sliced (reserved for garnish)

1. Mix all piquant marinade ingredients together.

2. Marinate sea bass and vegetables 20–30 minutes in large shallow baking dish.

3. Preheat grill. Place sea bass and vegetables directly on grill. Grill with lid down (roast) 10 minutes on each side.

4. Plate in decorative fashion with fresh herbs and lemon slices for garnish.

## Cook's Tip

*A large grill pan can also be used in place of an outdoor grill if you don't have access to one.*

**EXCHANGES/CHOICES: 4 VEGETABLE, 3 LEAN MEAT, 1 FAT**
**CALORIES 285, CALORIES FROM FAT 100,**
**TOTAL FAT 11 G, SATURATED FAT 1.2 G, TRANS FAT 0 G,**
**CHOLESTEROL 45 MG, SODIUM 325 MG, TOTAL CARBOHYDRATE 24 G,**
**DIETARY FIBER 7 G, SUGARS 10 G, PROTEIN 24 G**

*Not only are the beans a healthy addition to this* **Halibut in Tomato Basil Broth***, they also help absorb some of the delicious broth so you don't miss a drop.*

**Serves 4 / Serving Size: 1/4 recipe**

# halibut in tomato basil broth

**2 tsp** extra virgin olive oil

**1 lb** halibut fillet

**1/4 tsp** fine sea salt

**1/4 tsp** freshly ground black pepper

**2 cloves** garlic, crushed and chopped

**4 cups** small white beans, drained and rinsed (two 15 oz cans)

**6** plum tomatoes, chopped (about 2 cups)

**1/2 cup** fresh basil leaves, torn

**1 Tbsp** fresh oregano leaves

**2 Tbsp** chopped fresh chives

**1 cup** white wine or chicken stock

**1 cup** chicken stock

1. Heat olive oil in large skillet and add fish. Sprinkle fish with salt and pepper and sprinkle garlic directly onto pan surface. Cook 3 minutes. Turn fish with a large pancake turner.

2. Add beans, tomatoes, basil, oregano, chives, wine, and stock. Cover. Cook until fish is tender and begins to flake, about 5 minutes.

3. Place in large bowl with plenty of the tomato basil broth. Serve with Sautéed Spinach & Garlic (see recipe on page 155).

## Cook's Tip

*Halibut can be pricey and is worth the money, but it is also seasonal. Nice thick pieces of cod are also great here.*

**EXCHANGES/CHOICES: 2 STARCH, 4 LEAN MEAT**
**CALORIES 355, CALORIES FROM FAT 55,**
**TOTAL FAT 6 G, SATURATED FAT 0.7 G, TRANS FAT 0 G,**
**CHOLESTEROL 35 MG, SODIUM 715 MG, TOTAL CARBOHYDRATE 36 G,**
**DIETARY FIBER 9 G, SUGARS 6 G, PROTEIN 35 G**

*The mushroom crust in this **Mushroom-Crusted Sea Bass** is a little different from what you might normally make, but it is ever so delicious!*

**Serves 4 / Serving Size: 1/4 recipe**

# mushroom-crusted sea bass

**5 oz** fresh mushrooms

**1 clove** garlic, peeled and crushed

**1/4 cup** parsley leaves

**1/2 cup** unseasoned, whole-grain bread crumbs

**1/4 tsp** salt

**1/4 tsp** freshly ground black pepper

**1 lb** Chilean sea bass, cut into 4 portions

**1 Tbsp** extra virgin olive oil

**2 Tbsp** chopped shallots (1 medium)

**2 plum** tomatoes chopped

**1 1/2 cups** white wine

1. Place mushrooms, garlic, and parsley in the food processor. Process until finely chopped. Add bread crumbs, salt, and pepper. Mix well. Mixture will be a fine paste. Coat one side of sea bass with mushroom mixture.

2. Place extra virgin olive oil in sauté pan and heat. Place fish, mushroom-coated side down, in the sauté pan and brown for about 2 minutes on medium to high heat. Turn fish.

3. Add shallots, plum tomatoes, remaining mushroom paste, and white wine. Bring to a boil and immediately reduce heat to low. Using a small wire whisk or a fork, blend mushroom paste into wine.

4. Cover pan and cook approximately 10 minutes or until fish is done. Place fish on dinner plate and spoon sauce around fish.

EXCHANGES/CHOICES: 1/2 STARCH, 1 VEGETABLE, 3 LEAN MEAT
CALORIES 230, CALORIES FROM FAT 55,
TOTAL FAT 6 G, SATURATED FAT 0.5 G, TRANS FAT 0 G,
CHOLESTEROL 45 MG, SODIUM 245 MG, TOTAL CARBOHYDRATE 12 G,
DIETARY FIBER 3 G, SUGARS 3 G, PROTEIN 24 G

*Phyllo dough has almost no fat so it's a nice alternative to a traditional pie crust dough. This **Phyllo-Crusted Pot Pie** is delicious and healthy.*

**Serves 8 / Serving Size: 1/8 recipe**

# phyllo-crusted pot pie

**2 lb** thick fish fillet, cut into bite-sized pieces (cod, snapper, or flounder)
**2 tsp** extra virgin olive oil
**1/2 cup** chopped onion
**1 clove** garlic, minced
**1 cup** celery, sliced 1/4-inch thick
**1 cup** carrot, sliced 1/4-inch thick
**2 Tbsp** unsalted butter

**1/4 cup** all-purpose flour
**2 cups** chicken stock
**1 cup** frozen baby peas
**2 Tbsp** chopped Italian parsley
**1/4 tsp** fine sea salt
**1/4 tsp** freshly ground pepper
**1 package** phyllo dough, defrosted in the refrigerator

1. Preheat oven to 375°.

2. Saute fish 2–3 minutes and set aside. Add olive oil, onion, and garlic and cook 2–3 minutes until they begin to soften. Add celery and carrot and cook 5 minutes. Set aside.

3. Melt butter in second saucepan. Over medium heat, whisk in flour and mix well. Gradually add 1 cup stock to saucepan. Cook 2–3 minutes until mixture begins to thicken and takes on a golden color.

4. Add fish, peas, parsley, and additional stock to achieve desired consistency. Add salt and pepper to taste. Place mixture in baking dish.

5. Unwrap phyllo dough, lay it on work surface, and cut into 1-inch strips. Toss the strips together and lay on top of pot pie. Bake at 375° for about 20 minutes or until phyllo is golden and pie is bubbly.

EXCHANGES/CHOICES: 3 STARCH, 3 LEAN MEAT
CALORIES 355, CALORIES FROM FAT 55,
TOTAL FAT 6 G, SATURATED FAT 2.4 G, TRANS FAT 0 G,
CHOLESTEROL 55 MG, SODIUM 585 MG, TOTAL CARBOHYDRATE 46 G,
DIETARY FIBER 3 G, SUGARS 3 G, PROTEIN 26 G

*Blueberries are considered a "superfruit" because they're full of antioxidants. This **Roasted Lemon Garlic Cod with Lemon Blueberry Salsa** is filled with 2 whole cups of blueberries, so it's nutritious and delicious.*

**Serves 4 / Serving Size: 1/4 recipe**

# roasted lemon garlic cod
## with lemon blueberry salsa

**lemon blueberry salsa**

**2 cups** fresh blueberries (frozen will also work)

**1/2 cup** thinly sliced celery (about 1 large or 2 medium stalks)

**3/4 cup** thinly sliced scallions (1 small bunch)

**1/2 cup** roughly chopped fresh Italian parsley

**2** lemons, juiced

**1 Tbsp** extra virgin olive oil

**1/4 tsp** fine sea salt

**1/4 tsp** black pepper

**1/4 tsp** ground ginger

---

**1 lb** thick cod fillet

**1** lemon, juiced

**1** clove garlic, minced

1. Preheat oven to 375°.

2. Mix all lemon blueberry salsa ingredients together and set aside while preparing cod.

3. Place cod on parchment-lined baking sheet and coat with lemon juice and garlic. Roast in preheated oven for 10–20 minutes or until fish is opaque all the way through.

4. Slice cod and serve with some of the salsa, a nice green salad or green beans, and couscous.

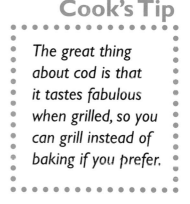

## Cook's Tip

*The great thing about cod is that it tastes fabulous when grilled, so you can grill instead of baking if you prefer.*

EXCHANGES/CHOICES: 1 FRUIT, 3 LEAN MEAT
CALORIES 185, CALORIES FROM FAT 40,
TOTAL FAT 4.5 G, SATURATED FAT 0.7 G, TRANS FAT 0 G,
CHOLESTEROL 50 MG, SODIUM 105 MG, TOTAL CARBOHYDRATE 16 G,
DIETARY FIBER 3 G, SUGARS 9 G, PROTEIN 22 G

*This **Snapper with Shallot, Basil & Garlic** recipe offers a colorful and delicious blend of both familiar and tasty ingredients.*

**Serves 4 / Serving Size: 1/4 recipe**

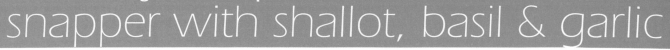

# snapper with shallot, basil & garlic

**1 lb** snapper fillet (or any large white fish fillet)

**1 tsp** fine sea salt

**1/4 tsp** freshly ground pepper

**1 Tbsp** extra virgin olive oil

**2** shallots, minced

**1 clove** garlic, minced

**4** small zucchini, 4–6 inches long, sliced into 1/4-inch rounds

**3/4 cup** dry white wine or chicken or fish stock

**2 cups** chopped very ripe plum tomatoes

**1/2 cup** fresh basil, chopped

1. Season fish with salt and pepper and refrigerate.

2. Place extra virgin olive oil in sauté pan. Sauté shallot and garlic until shallot starts to become translucent. Add zucchini and sauté 1–2 minutes. Remove from pan.

3. Add snapper and sauté on each side. Add white wine or stock. Cover and simmer until fish is done. This will vary depending on the thickness of your fish. Use 10 minutes per inch of thickness.

4. Return zucchini mixture to pan and add the chopped tomatoes and fresh basil. Heat thoroughly. Serve with pasta, rice, couscous, or whole-grain crusty Italian bread.

## Cook's Tip

*Shallots are an elegant but mild alternative to onions and garlic; however, you can use a little onion and garlic combined if you don't have shallots at home.*

**EXCHANGES/CHOICES: 2 VEGETABLE, 3 LEAN MEAT**
**CALORIES 200, CALORIES FROM FAT 45,**
**TOTAL FAT 5 G, SATURATED FAT 0.8 G, TRANS FAT 0 G,**
**CHOLESTEROL 40 MG, SODIUM 660 MG, TOTAL CARBOHYDRATE 11 G,**
**DIETARY FIBER 3 G, SUGARS 5 G, PROTEIN 26 G**

*Using the flavored skewers for these* **Thai Fish Kabobs** *makes it even more tasty, but regular skewers will also work if that's all you have.*

**Serves 4 / Serving Size: 1/4 recipe**
# thai fish kabobs

**1 lb** thick white fish fillets (Chilean sea bass or cod), cut into 8–12 pieces

**1 package** Thai coconut lime skewers

**1 tsp** canola oil

**1/2 cup** chicken stock

**2 Tbsp** light coconut milk

**2 Tbsp** lime juice (1 lime)

**1 cup** snow peas, julienned

**1 cup** matchstick carrots

**1/2 cup** cilantro leaves, roughly chopped

1. Thread fish cubes on four Thai coconut lime skewers and let sit for 15 minutes.

2. Coat sauté pan with canola oil and heat. Add skewers to heated pan. Sauté skewers on one side for 1 minute. Using tongs, turn skewers to brown opposite side.

3. Immediately add chicken stock, coconut milk, lime juice, snow peas, carrots, and cilantro to pan. Bring to a boil, reduce heat to low, and simmer covered for 5 minutes.

4. Serve with jasmine rice.

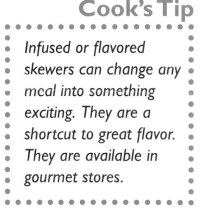

## Cook's Tip

*Infused or flavored skewers can change any meal into something exciting. They are a shortcut to great flavor. They are available in gourmet stores.*

**EXCHANGES/CHOICES: 1 VEGETABLE, 3 LEAN MEAT**
**CALORIES 155, CALORIES FROM FAT 35,**
**TOTAL FAT 4 G, SATURATED FAT 0.4 G, TRANS FAT 0 G,**
**CHOLESTEROL 45 MG, SODIUM 225 MG, TOTAL CARBOHYDRATE 6 G,**
**DIETARY FIBER 2 G, SUGARS 3 G, PROTEIN 23 G**

*In this delightful **Tilapia Spinach Rolls** recipe, I am using Grana Padano cheese, which is a high-protein, full-flavored Italian cheese.*

**Serves 4 / Serving Size: 1/4 recipe**

# tilapia spinach rolls

**1 lb** tilapia fillet, cut into 4 pieces

**1/4 tsp** fine sea salt

**1/4 tsp** freshly ground pepper

**16 leaves** baby spinach (4 leaves per fillet)

**1/4 cup** grated Grana Padano cheese

**1 cup** dry white wine

**1/2 cup** chicken or vegetable stock

**1** shallot, minced

**3/4 cup** slivered almonds

**8 medium slices** tomato

**1 1/3 cups** cooked brown rice

1. Preheat oven to 375°.

2. Lay fillets out on work surface. Season lightly with salt and pepper. Lay several spinach leaves on top of each fillet. Sprinkle with Grana Padano. Roll each fillet and secure with toothpick.

3. Place fillets in baking dish and surround them with white wine and stock. Sprinkle with minced shallot and almonds. Cover and bake 20 minutes. Uncover and cook 10 minutes more.

4. Serve each fillet with 2 slices of tomato and 1/3 cup brown rice.

## Cook's Tip

*If tomatoes are out of season, chopped cherry tomatoes would make a good choice, substituting for the larger, slicing tomatoes.*

**EXCHANGES/CHOICES: 1 STARCH, 1/2 CARBOHYDRATE, 4 LEAN MEAT, 2 FAT**
**CALORIES 380, CALORIES FROM FAT 160,**
**TOTAL FAT 18 G, SATURATED FAT 3.4 G, TRANS FAT 0 G,**
**CHOLESTEROL 85 MG, SODIUM 355 MG, TOTAL CARBOHYDRATE 23 G,**
**DIETARY FIBER 5 G, SUGARS 3 G, PROTEIN 32 G**

# Chapter 7:

# SHELLFISH

*The "cream" sauce in this* **Baked Scallops & Mushroom**

**Sauce** *recipe is low-fat and blends perfectly with the scallops.*

**Serves 4 / Serving Size: 1/4 recipe**

# baked scallops & mushroom sauce

**1 Tbsp** extra virgin olive oil

**1 1/2 lb** mixed mushrooms, roughly chopped

**2 Tbsp** minced shallots (about 1 large)

**1/2 cup** fresh basil, chopped

**1/2 cup** flat Italian parsley, chopped

**1/2 cup** dry white wine or chicken stock

**1 cup** evaporated skim milk

**1/4 tsp** fine sea salt

**1/8 tsp** freshly ground white pepper

**12 oz** bay scallops, rinsed

1. Preheat oven to 400°.

2. Heat a large sauté pan and add the olive oil, mushrooms, and shallots. Cook until mushrooms begin to wilt and shallots begin to become translucent, about 3–4 minutes.

3. Add herbs, wine, or stock, evaporated skim milk, salt, and pepper. Bring to boil and immediately turn to low. Add scallops and coat well with sauce. Transfer scallops to baking dish. Bake 20 minutes. Serve immediately.

4. Garnish with additional chopped fresh herbs.

## Cook's Tip

*If you have "shell" baking dishes, you can make great use of them here, but any nice dish will do.*

**EXCHANGES/CHOICES:** 1/2 **FAT-FREE MILK,** 1 **VEGETABLE,** 3 **LEAN MEAT**
**CALORIES** 200, **CALORIES FROM FAT** 45,
**TOTAL FAT** 5 G, **SATURATED FAT** 0.7 G, **TRANS FAT** 0 G,
**CHOLESTEROL** 35 MG, **SODIUM** 400 MG, **TOTAL CARBOHYDRATE** 14 G,
**DIETARY FIBER** 2 G, **SUGARS** 10 G, **PROTEIN** 25 G

This **Bloody Mary Shrimp** is a versatile recipe that can be cooked on the grill or roasted in your oven. It's even a great idea to keep peeled, deveined shrimp in your freezer so you're prepared for a quick meal.

**Serves 4 / Serving Size: 1/4 recipe**

# bloody mary shrimp

**1 lb** large shrimp, peeled and deveined

**1 cup** tomato juice

**1/4 cup** roughly chopped Italian parsley

**3 cloves** garlic, sliced into rounds

**1/2 tsp** celery seed

**1 oz** vodka

**1 1/2 tsp** low-sodium Worcestershire sauce

**1** lemon, juiced

**1 1/2 tsp** prepared horseradish

**1/4 tsp** freshly ground mixed peppercorns

1. Defrost shrimp by running under cold water. Do not use hot water as it will change the texture of the shrimp.

2. Mix together tomato juice, parsley, garlic, celery seed, vodka, Worcestershire, lemon juice, horseradish, and pepper. Marinate shrimp for a minimum of 20 minutes or up to 2 hours.

3. Soak wooden skewers in cold water for at least 20 minutes. This will help prevent charring. Preheat grill. Brush grill to ensure clean surface. Thread shrimp on skewers and grill until they turn pink, about 3 minutes on each side for large shrimp.

4. Serve with couscous cooked in chicken stock or small pasta, such as orzo.

## Cook's Tip

*If broiling, preheat broiler prior to placing shrimp in the oven. If roasting, preheat oven to 400°. Broiling will take about 3 minutes per side and roasting will take about 10 minutes.*

**EXCHANGES/CHOICES: 3 LEAN MEAT**
**CALORIES 130, CALORIES FROM FAT 10,**
**TOTAL FAT 1 G, SATURATED FAT 0.3 G, TRANS FAT 0 G,**
**CHOLESTEROL 185 MG, SODIUM 415 MG, TOTAL CARBOHYDRATE 3 G,**
**DIETARY FIBER 0 G, SUGARS 1 G, PROTEIN 25 G**

*Quick and simple—but these* **Crab Lettuce Wraps** *don't taste it or look it! Lump crabmeat is costly, so claw or backfin work well for less money.*

**Serves 3 / Serving Size: I wrap**

# crab lettuce wraps

**8 oz** pasteurized crabmeat

**3** large lettuce leaves (Boston or Bibb lettuce works well)

**3 tsp** Asian peanut sauce

**3 tsp** julienned or matchstick carrots

**6 slices** cucumber, sliced paper thin

**1 (4 oz) package** sprouts

1. Open crabmeat and place in a bowl. Look through for any cartilage or shell.

2. Begin by laying a piece of lettuce on a plate. Top with crab, peanut sauce, carrots, and sprouts. Roll to enclose filling.

## Cook's Tip

*A sharp knife is your friend, and will do the work for you, especially when paper-thin slices are desired, as they are in this recipe.*

**EXCHANGES/CHOICES: 2 LEAN MEAT**
**CALORIES 75, CALORIES FROM FAT 15,**
**TOTAL FAT 1.5 G, SATURATED FAT 0.2 G, TRANS FAT 0 G,**
**CHOLESTEROL 105 MG, SODIUM 375 MG, TOTAL CARBOHYDRATE 1 G,**
**DIETARY FIBER 0 G, SUGARS 1 G, PROTEIN 14 G**

*This delicious Crab-Stuffed Portobello Mushrooms recipe serves as an elegant first course or light lunch.*

**Serves 4 / Serving Size: 1/4 recipe**

# crab-stuffed portobello mushrooms

**12 oz** pasteurized lump crabmeat

**2** lemons, juiced (divided use)

**4** portobello mushroom caps

**1 Tbsp, plus 1 tsp** extra virgin olive oil

**2 cups** mixed spring greens

**1/8 tsp** fine sea salt

**1/8 tsp** black pepper

1. Mix crab and half of the lemon juice.

2. Clean mushrooms. Remove gills with spoon. Brush with olive oil. Grill 3–4 minutes on each side, or until tender when pierced with a fork.

3. Place mixed greens in bowl. Mix olive oil with remaining lemon juice. Add salt and pepper. Toss well.

4. Place 1 mushroom cap on a plate, top with 1/4 of the salad greens, and 3 oz of crab.

## Cook's Tip

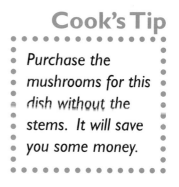

*Purchase the mushrooms for this dish without the stems. It will save you some money.*

EXCHANGES/CHOICES: 2 LEAN MEAT, 1/2 FAT
CALORIES 125, CALORIES FROM FAT 55,
TOTAL FAT 6 G, SATURATED FAT 0.8 G, TRANS FAT 0 G,
CHOLESTEROL 115 MG, SODIUM 425 MG, TOTAL CARBOHYDRATE 3 G,
DIETARY FIBER 1 G, SUGARS 1 G, PROTEIN 16 G

*This **Mexi-Scallops** dish is full of Mexican flavor but is super easy and fast to prepare, so you can make it anytime you're craving Mexican.*

**Serves 4 / Serving Size: 1/4 recipe**

# mexi-scallops

**1 lb** frozen bay scallops, thawed

**1 (10 oz) can** diced tomatoes with green chilies

**1/4 cup** minced onion (1 small)

**3 Tbsp** sliced black olives

**1 cup** frozen corn

**1/2 cup** frozen baby lima beans

**1/2 tsp** ground cumin

**1 cup** cilantro leaves, roughly chopped

**1 Tbsp** cornmeal

**2 oz** reduced-fat cheddar cheese, grated (divided use)

1. Preheat oven to 425°.

2. Combine all ingredients except the cheddar cheese in a large mixing bowl. Stir. Add 1 oz of the cheddar cheese and stir. Pour contents into a baking dish. Top with remaining 1 oz of cheddar cheese. Bake at 450° for 15 minutes.

3. Serve with brown rice.

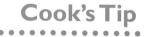

## Cook's Tip

*Frozen scallops will work in this dish, but be sure to thaw them before cooking. The bay scallops are the small scallops. I remember this because the bay is smaller than the sea.*

**EXCHANGES/CHOICES: 1 STARCH, 1 VEGETABLE, 3 LEAN MEAT
CALORIES 225, CALORIES FROM FAT 55,
TOTAL FAT 6 G, SATURATED FAT 2.1 G, TRANS FAT 0 G,
CHOLESTEROL 55 MG, SODIUM 695 MG, TOTAL CARBOHYDRATE 18 G,
DIETARY FIBER 3 G, SUGARS 4 G, PROTEIN 27 G**

*Enjoy a light meal of steamed mussels without leaving home
with this **Mussels with Lemon and Garlic Dip** dish.*

**Serves 2 / Serving Size:1/2 recipe**

# mussels with lemon and garlic dip

**4 large stems** fresh basil (with leaves)

**4 large stems** fresh oregano (with leaves)

**3** lemons, sliced

**1/4 tsp** sea salt

**1/4 tsp** freshly ground pepper

**2 lb** mussels or 2 dozen cherrystone clams, scrubbed

**2 cups** dry white wine (Orvieto or Pinot Grigio)

1. Layer herbs, lemon, salt, pepper, mussels, and wine in a chef's pan.
   Cover.  Bring to a boil and steam until mussels/clams open.

2. Serve in bowls with crusty Italian bread and extra broth.

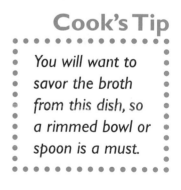

## Cook's Tip

*You will want to
savor the broth
from this dish, so
a rimmed bowl or
spoon is a must.*

**EXCHANGES/CHOICES: 1/2 CARBOHYDRATE, 2 LEAN MEAT, 2 FAT
CALORIES 235, CALORIES FROM FAT 80,
TOTAL FAT 9 G, SATURATED FAT 0.9 G, TRANS FAT 0 G,
CHOLESTEROL 30 MG, SODIUM 410 MG, TOTAL CARBOHYDRATE 9 G,
DIETARY FIBER 0 G, SUGARS 6 G, PROTEIN 14 G**

*Why go out to dinner when you can create a beautiful dish like these **Pasta Nests with White Clam Sauce** at home?*

**Serves 4 / Serving Size: 1/4 recipe**

# pasta nests with white clam sauce

- **1 Tbsp** extra virgin olive oil
- **12–16 oz** fettuccine or tagliatelle pasta nests (see Cook's Tip)
- **2 cloves** garlic, minced
- **1 cup** fresh basil leaves, chopped (additional for garnish)
- **1/4 cup** fresh oregano leaves, chopped (additional for garnish)
- **1/4 cup** Italian parsley, chopped (additional for garnish)
- **1 1/2 cups** dry white wine
- **2 (10 oz) cans** baby clams
- **3 cups** water
- **2 cups** clam juice or chicken stock
- **1/4 cup** freshly squeezed lemon juice
- **1/4 tsp** fine sea salt
- **1/2 tsp** black pepper

1. Place olive oil in a sauté pan. Heat to medium and add pasta nests. Cook pasta until golden on first side. Turn. Add garlic and herbs in between nests and cook until fragrant, about 1 minute.

2. Add wine, canned clams, water, clam juice or stock, lemon juice, salt, and pepper. Liquid should cover pasta. Cover and cook 6–10 minutes or until pasta is al dente.

3. Garnish with additional fresh herbs, if desired.

## Cook's Tip

*Pasta nests come in many sizes so you have to use your judgment in determining how many to use. A good guideline is to use enough to comfortably fill the pan without crowding. Most pasta nests are about 1 oz each.*

**EXCHANGES/CHOICES: 4 1/2 STARCH, 3 LEAN MEAT**
**CALORIES 485, CALORIES FROM FAT 55,**
**TOTAL FAT 6 G, SATURATED FAT 0.7 G, TRANS FAT 0 G,**
**CHOLESTEROL 45 MG, SODIUM 500 MG, TOTAL CARBOHYDRATE 70 G,**
**DIETARY FIBER 3 G, SUGARS 7 G, PROTEIN 28 G**

*There are some restaurant dishes that are so easy, we can make them at home—this* **Pasta with Diced Tomato and Zucchini** *is one of them.*

**Serves 4 / Serving Size: 1/4 recipe**

# pasta with diced tomato & zucchini

**8 oz** uncooked spaghetti, penne, or rotini

**2 tsp** extra virgin olive oil

**2 cloves** garlic, minced

**12 oz** medium shrimp, peeled and deveined

**2** medium zucchini, quartered and sliced 1/4-inch thick

**6–8** large, ripe plum tomatoes

**1/4 tsp** fine sea salt

**1/8 tsp** freshly ground pepper

**1 cup** chicken or vegetable stock

**1 cup** fresh basil, chopped

1. Cook pasta to al dente stage, approximately 8–10 minutes. While pasta is cooking, start the sauce.

2. Thinly film a sauté pan with olive oil. Add garlic and cook until fragrant. Add shrimp and zucchini. Sauté until shrimp are pink and opaque in the center, about 3–4 minutes.

3. Add tomatoes and toss with shrimp and zucchini. Season with sea salt and pepper. Add stock and basil. Heat thoroughly. Add cooked pasta to sauce. Mix well.

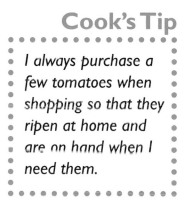

## Cook's Tip

*I always purchase a few tomatoes when shopping so that they ripen at home and are on hand when I need them.*

**EXCHANGES/CHOICES:** 2 1/2 STARCH, 2 VEGETABLE, 2 LEAN MEAT
CALORIES 345, CALORIES FROM FAT 40,
TOTAL FAT 4.5 G, SATURATED FAT 0.7 G, TRANS FAT 0 G,
CHOLESTEROL 90 MG, SODIUM 555 MG, TOTAL CARBOHYDRATE 54 G,
DIETARY FIBER 6 G, SUGARS 8 G, PROTEIN 22 G

*This **Risotto with Shrimp & Lemon** dish must be served immediately. It is best when it's fresh out of the oven.*

**Serves 4 / Serving Size: 1/4 recipe**

# risotto with shrimp & lemon

**5 cups** no-salt-added, low-fat chicken broth

**1** lemon, juiced

**2 Tbsp** extra virgin olive oil

**4 Tbsp** fresh chopped chives (divided use)

**1 1/2 cups** carnaroli or arborio rice, checked over for imperfect grains

**1/8 tsp** fine sea salt

**1/2 tsp** freshly ground pepper

**1 lb** large, peeled, deveined shrimp

**2 oz** freshly grated Parmigiano-Reggiano

1. Bring broth and lemon juice to a boil in 4-quart saucepan. Keep simmering on stove.

2. Using a heavy 4-quart saucepan or chef's pan, thinly film the pan with olive oil and add 2 Tbsp chives. Sauté until chives release aroma.

3. Add rice, salt, and pepper and coat rice grains with olive oil mixture. Add broth mixture 1 cup at a time and stir until liquid is absorbed. This takes time and patience, at least 30 minutes.

4. After last addition of stock, add shrimp, and steam until pink. Add Parmigiano-Reggiano. Stir well. Garnish with 2 Tbsp chives. Serve immediately.

## Cook's Tip

*Adding hot liquid to risotto makes a world of difference. It helps to create the "creaminess."*

EXCHANGES/CHOICES: 3 1/2 STARCH, 4 LEAN MEAT, 1/2 FAT
CALORIES 465, CALORIES FROM FAT 115,
TOTAL FAT 13 G, SATURATED FAT 4 G, TRANS FAT 0 G,
CHOLESTEROL 170 MG, SODIUM 540 MG, TOTAL CARBOHYDRATE 51 G,
DIETARY FIBER 2 G, SUGARS 1 G, PROTEIN 33 G

*When tomatoes are out of season, you can't go wrong keeping a container of cherry or grape tomatoes in the house for a quick "relish." The relish in this **Scallops with Cherry Tomato Relish** is a perfect example.*

**Serves 4 / Serving Size: 1/4 recipe**

# scallops with cherry tomato relish

**1 Tbsp** extra virgin olive oil

**4 cloves** garlic, crushed and skin removed

**1 lb** large sea scallops

**1 pint** cherry tomatoes

**1/4 tsp** fine sea salt

**1/4 tsp** freshly ground black pepper

**1/4 cup** fresh basil leaves

**1/2 cup** dry white wine

1. Place oil and crushed garlic in large sauté pan. Heat until garlic becomes fragrant and begins to brown. Once it begins to brown, remove from the oil. Set aside.

2. Add scallops and cook until golden on first side, approximately 3 minutes. Turn and cook until golden on second side, which will take about 3 minutes.

3. While scallops are cooking on second side, add sliced cherry tomatoes, salt, and pepper. Cook until tomatoes are soft, about 3 minutes. Add basil leaves and wine. Cook 1 minute, stirring to blend tomatoes and basil.

4. Serve with whole-grain pasta with Pesto (see recipe on page 142).

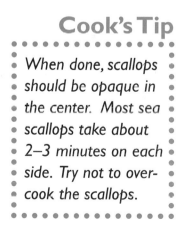

## Cook's Tip

*When done, scallops should be opaque in the center. Most sea scallops take about 2–3 minutes on each side. Try not to over-cook the scallops.*

EXCHANGES/CHOICES: 1 VEGETABLE, 3 LEAN MEAT
CALORIES 155, CALORIES FROM FAT 40,
TOTAL FAT 4.5 G, SATURATED FAT 0.6 G, TRANS FAT 0 G,
CHOLESTEROL 45 MG, SODIUM 380 MG, TOTAL CARBOHYDRATE 4 G,
DIETARY FIBER 1 G, SUGARS 2 G, PROTEIN 21 G

*Baby spinach has to be one of the best things to happen to a grocery store in a long time, because it's healthy and easy to add to anything. It adds a deliciously light touch to this* **Sea Scallops with Baby Spinach** *dish.*

**Serves 4 / Serving Size: 1/4 recipe**

# sea scallops with baby spinach

**1 (9 oz) bag** baby spinach
**1 Tbsp** extra virgin olive oil
**12 oz** sea scallops
**1/2 cup** dry white wine
**1** lemon, juiced
**1/4 tsp** fine sea salt
**1/8 tsp** freshly ground black pepper

1. Rinse the spinach in a large colander. Place directly into sauté pan and cook until spinach wilts (do not add any oil or butter to the pan, cook in just the water left from rinsing). Place on serving plates.

2. In the meantime, thinly film sauté pan with olive oil and heat to medium-high. Pat the scallops dry. Add scallops to pan and sear first side. Turn scallops and brown other side. Place scallops on top of spinach.

3. Add white wine, lemon juice, salt, and pepper to scallops pan. The addition of the wine will deglaze the pan and release any bits that are sticking. This will create a nice light sauce. Sprinkle the scallops and spinach with the sauce.

EXCHANGES/CHOICES: 2 LEAN MEAT, 1/2 FAT
CALORIES 130, CALORIES FROM FAT 40,
TOTAL FAT 4.5 G, SATURATED FAT 0.6 G, TRANS FAT 0 G,
CHOLESTEROL 35 MG, SODIUM 370 MG, TOTAL CARBOHYDRATE 3 G,
DIETARY FIBER 1 G, SUGARS 1 G, PROTEIN 17 G

*This **Sea Scallops with Lemon & Herbs** dish is always a big hit in my cooking classes and I have received countless emails telling me how often my students serve it in their own homes.*

**Serves 4 / Serving Size: 1/4 recipe**

# sea scallops with lemon & herbs

**12 oz** uncooked whole-grain linguine

**2 cloves** garlic, sliced thin

**2 Tbsp** extra virgin olive oil

**1/2 cup** roughly chopped fresh herbs (Italian parsley, basil, chives)

**1/4 tsp** freshly ground black pepper

**1/4 tsp** fine sea salt

**2** lemons, juiced

**12 oz** sea scallops, rinsed

1. Cook pasta to al dente stage, approximately 8–10 minutes. While pasta is cooking, start the sauce.

2. Slice garlic and place in sauté pan. Add oil and heat until fragrant and garlic is light to golden brown. Transfer to heat-proof bowl. Add herbs, salt, pepper, and lemon juice. Whisk together until creamy. Toss with pasta.

3. Re-heat sauté pan and add scallops. Sear on first side for about 2 minutes. Turn and sear on second side.

4. Place scallops on top of pasta with lemon garlic sauce. Sprinkle with fresh herbs. Additional fresh herbs and lemon slices can be used for garnish.

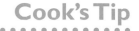

## Cook's Tip

*Fresh lemon juice is a must, so please don't use bottled lemon juice or anything that's not fresh squeezed.*

EXCHANGES/CHOICES: 4 STARCH, 3 LEAN MEAT
CALORIES 455, CALORIES FROM FAT 80,
TOTAL FAT 9 G, SATURATED FAT 1.2 G, TRANS FAT 0 G,
CHOLESTEROL 35 MG, SODIUM 330 MG, TOTAL CARBOHYDRATE 63 G,
DIETARY FIBER 9 G, SUGARS 2 G, PROTEIN 29 G

*Jasmine rice, shrimp, and healthful ginger team up to create this delicious and guilt-free* **Shrimp & Asparagus Stir-fry** *dish.*

**Serves 4 / Serving Size: 1/4 recipe**

# shrimp & asparagus stir-fry

**1 cup** uncooked jasmine rice
**1 (2-inch) piece** fresh ginger, cut into 1/2-inch slices
**12 oz** medium shrimp, peeled and deveined
**1 cup** white wine
**1 Tbsp** fish sauce
**1 Tbsp** cornstarch
**1 cup** fish stock or clam juice
**2 Tbsp** canola oil
**2–3 cloves** garlic, peeled and sliced
**1 (1-inch) piece** ginger, peeled and sliced
**1 lb** fresh asparagus, cut into 2-inch pieces

1. Place rice, 2 cups water, and ginger in 4-quart saucepan. Cover and bring to boil. When you see steam, turn pan to low and cook about 20 minutes. Remove ginger to serve.

2. In a medium-sized bowl, marinate shrimp in white wine and fish sauce. Mix in cornstarch and fish stock.

3. Heat oil in a large sauté pan, chef's pan, or wok. Add garlic and ginger and cook until golden. Remove. Add asparagus and cook until crisp tender. Push to side of pan. Drain shrimp and reserve marinade. Add shrimp to pan and cook until pink.

4. Mix reserved marinade with cornstarch mixture and add to stir-fry. Cook until sauce is thickened. Serve over ginger rice.

**EXCHANGES/CHOICES: 2 1/2 STARCH, 1 VEGETABLE, 2 LEAN MEAT, 1/2 FAT**
**CALORIES 345, CALORIES FROM FAT 70,**
**TOTAL FAT 8 G, SATURATED FAT 0.7 G, TRANS FAT 0 G,**
**CHOLESTEROL 90 MG, SODIUM 595 MG, TOTAL CARBOHYDRATE 44 G,**
**DIETARY FIBER 2 G, SUGARS 2 G, PROTEIN 18 G**

*With or without the pasta, this* **Shrimp, Baby Spinach & Pignoli** *recipe has a great combination of delicious flavors that blend together perfectly.*

**Serves 4 / Serving Size: 1/4 recipe**

# shrimp, baby spinach & pignoli

**1/2 cup** pignoli (pine nuts)

**1 Tbsp** extra virgin olive oil

**12 oz** large shrimp, peeled and deveined

**2 cloves** garlic, minced

**9 oz** baby spinach (1 large bag)

**1 cup** chicken stock

**12 oz** cooked whole-grain pasta (penne or rotelle)

**1/4 cup** grated asiago cheese

1. Place pignoli in a dry skillet in a single layer and stir over medium-high heat until golden. Immediately remove from pan to prevent further browning.

2. Thinly film the sauté pan with extra virgin olive oil. Add shrimp. Toss well to coat with olive oil. Add garlic and cook until shrimp begin to turn pink.

3. Add spinach and stock and cover pan. Cook until spinach is wilted. When spinach is wilted, add cooked pasta and toss well. Sprinkle with grated asiago and toasted pignoli.

## Cook's Tip

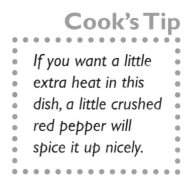

*If you want a little extra heat in this dish, a little crushed red pepper will spice it up nicely.*

**EXCHANGES/CHOICES: 2 STARCH, 1 VEGETABLE, 2 LEAN MEAT, 3 FAT**
**CALORIES 405, CALORIES FROM FAT 170,**
**TOTAL FAT 19 G, SATURATED FAT 3 G, TRANS FAT 0 G,**
**CHOLESTEROL 95 MG, SODIUM 525 MG, TOTAL CARBOHYDRATE 39 G,**
**DIETARY FIBER 7 G, SUGARS 3 G, PROTEIN 23 G**

*This **Shrimp Quesadilla** recipe was inspired by a cooking class I took in Arizona. I'm sure you will love it as much as I do.*

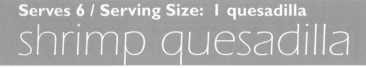

# shrimp quesadilla

**12 oz** uncooked medium shrimp, peeled, deveined, and cut in half lengthwise
**1 clove** garlic, minced
**1 Tbsp** canola oil
**6 (6-inch)** flour tortillas
**2 tsp** fresh Cilantro and Sun-Flower Seed Pesto (see recipe on page **140**)
**1 cup** fat-free cheddar cheese
Canola oil spray

1. Preheat oven to 375°.

2. Preheat large sauté pan to medium-high heat. Toss shrimp and garlic with 1 Tbsp oil. Add shrimp to pan and sauté for about 2 minutes. Transfer to bowl.

3. Lay flour tortillas out flat and layer each on one half with some sautéed shrimp, 2 tsp of Cilantro and Sun-Flower Seed Pesto (recipe on page 140) and then cheese.

4. Fold tortillas in half and spray with olive oil cooking spray or your own canola oil. Bake in the oven for 10 minutes or until golden brown. Remove from pan. Cut it into wedges and drizzle pesto over all.

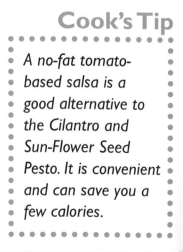

## Cook's Tip

*A no-fat tomato-based salsa is a good alternative to the Cilantro and Sun-Flower Seed Pesto. It is convenient and can save you a few calories.*

**EXCHANGES/CHOICES: 1 STARCH, 2 LEAN MEAT, 1 FAT
CALORIES 225, CALORIES FROM FAT 80,
TOTAL FAT 9 G, SATURATED FAT 1.2 G, TRANS FAT 0 G,
CHOLESTEROL 60 MG, SODIUM 475 MG, TOTAL CARBOHYDRATE 18 G,
DIETARY FIBER 2 G, SUGARS 1 G, PROTEIN 18 G**

*This delightful **Shrimp with Garlic** recipe was created to replicate a favorite dish served in the Cichetti bars in Venice, Italy.*

## Serves 4 / Serving Size: 1/4 recipe
# shrimp with garlic

**1 lb** of small shrimp, peeled and deveined
**1** large lemon, juiced
**2 cloves** garlic
**1 Tbsp** extra virgin olive oil
**1 cup** chopped fresh parsley
**1/4 tsp** fine sea salt

1. Bring a 4-quart pot filled with water to a boil. Boil the shrimp until they are pink outside and opaque inside, approximately 3 minutes. Remove from pot with slotted spoon.

2. Toss with lemon juice, garlic, extra virgin olive oil, parsley, and salt.

3. Serve with cooked polenta or top a green salad with this mixture.

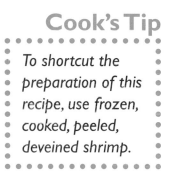

## Cook's Tip

*To shortcut the preparation of this recipe, use frozen, cooked, peeled, deveined shrimp.*

EXCHANGES/CHOICES: 2 LEAN MEAT
CALORIES 105, CALORIES FROM FAT 40,
TOTAL FAT 4.5 G, SATURATED FAT 0.7 G, TRANS FAT 0 G,
CHOLESTEROL 130 MG, SODIUM 310 MG, TOTAL CARBOHYDRATE 2 G,
DIETARY FIBER 1 G, SUGARS 0 G, PROTEIN 15 G

# Chapter 8:

# WHOLE FISH

*Fennel, tomato, and basil are another perfect combination that we don't use often enough. Their flavors blend together perfectly in this **Baked Whole Fish with Fennel, Tomato & Basil** recipe.*

**Serves 4 / Serving Size: 1/4 recipe**

# baked whole fish
## with fennel, tomato & basil

**1** fennel bulb (about 1 lb)
**6** plum tomatoes, very ripe
**1/2 cup** fresh basil leaves
**1/2 cup** fresh Italian parsley
**1 clove** garlic, minced
**1/2 tsp** fine sea salt
**1/2 tsp** freshly ground black pepper
**1** whole fish (trout, branzino, snapper), cleaned (gutted)
     with head and tail attached (about 1 1/2 to 2 lb)

1. Preheat oven to 400°.

2. Slice fennel from tip to core as thinly as possible. Chop plum tomatoes. Mix fennel, tomatoes, basil, parsley, garlic, salt, and pepper together. Spread three quarters of this mixture in a baking dish. Lay fish on top and top with remaining mixture.

3. Bake for 20 minutes until vegetables are tender and fish flakes with a fork. Cover with aluminum foil and let fish rest for 10 minutes before serving.

4. Serve with Orzo Pilaf (see recipe on page 154).

EXCHANGES/CHOICES: 2 VEGETABLE, 3 LEAN MEAT
CALORIES 160, CALORIES FROM FAT 20,
TOTAL FAT 2 G, SATURATED FAT 0.4 G, TRANS FAT 0 G,
CHOLESTEROL 45 MG, SODIUM 390 MG, TOTAL CARBOHYDRATE 9 G,
DIETARY FIBER 3 G, SUGARS 4 G, PROTEIN 27 G

*This **Grilled Whole Fish with Herbs** recipe is perfect for a fresh summer family dinner on the back deck or porch.*

**Serves 4 / Serving Size: 1/4 recipe**

# grilled whole fish with herbs

**1 cup** basil leaves

**1/2 cup** fresh Italian parsley leaves

**4 cloves** garlic, minced

**1** whole fish (trout, branzino, snapper), cleaned (gutted) with head and tail attached (about 1 1/2 to 2 lb)

**4 sprigs** fresh rosemary

**2 tsp** extra virgin olive oil

**1/4 tsp** fine sea salt

**1/4 tsp** freshly ground black pepper

**1/2 cup** dry white wine (Orvieto or Pinot Grigio)

1. Preheat grill to high.

2. Mix basil, parsley, and garlic together. Stuff fish with basil, parsley, and garlic. Add rosemary. Press to close. Rub gently with extra virgin olive oil and season with salt and pepper.

3. Tear off a piece of aluminum foil large enough to wrap the whole fish in. Place the stuffed fish on the foil and pour the white wine over it. Wrap tightly and place on preheated grill for 20–25 minutes or until fish flakes with a fork.

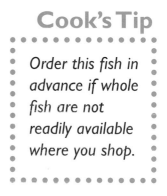

**Cook's Tip**

*Order this fish in advance if whole fish are not readily available where you shop.*

**EXCHANGES/CHOICES: 4 LEAN MEAT**
**CALORIES 160, CALORIES FROM FAT 35,**
**TOTAL FAT 4 G, SATURATED FAT 0.7 G, TRANS FAT 0 G,**
**CHOLESTEROL 45 MG, SODIUM 205 MG, TOTAL CARBOHYDRATE 2 G,**
**DIETARY FIBER 1 G, SUGARS 0 G, PROTEIN 26 G**

*This **Roasted Trout with Garlic & Lemon** would be a great meal after a day of trout fishing on your favorite lake.*

**Serves 4 / Serving Size: 1/4 recipe**

# roasted trout with garlic & lemon

**1/2 cup** fresh basil leaves

**1/4 cup** fresh rosemary

**1/2 cup** fresh Italian parsley

**3 cloves** garlic, sliced into rounds

**1** whole trout, cleaned (gutted) with head and tail attached (about 1 1/2 to 2 lb)

**2** preserved lemons, thinly sliced with seeds removed, or fresh lemons tossed with 1/2 tsp salt

Vegetable cooking spray

**1/2 tsp** black pepper

1. Preheat oven to 375°.

2. Remove basil, rosemary, and parsley from their stems.  Mix with garlic rounds in a small bowl.

3. Cut a pocket in the trout and tuck lemons, basil, parsley, and garlic inside.  Lightly spray the outside of the fish with vegetable cooking spray.  Sprinkle with pepper.

4. Place on a parchment-lined baking sheet and roast until the skin is nicely browned, about 30 minutes.

## Cook's Tip

*Preserved lemons can be purchased in your favorite gourmet store and will keep in the refrigerator for several months.*

EXCHANGES/CHOICES: 1/2 CARBOHYDRATE, 4 LEAN MEAT, 1 FAT
CALORIES 240, CALORIES FROM FAT 100,
TOTAL FAT 11 G, SATURATED FAT 1.9 G, TRANS FAT 0 G,
CHOLESTEROL 75 MG, SODIUM 370 MG, TOTAL CARBOHYDRATE 9 G,
DIETARY FIBER 3 G, SUGARS 2 G, PROTEIN 29 G

*Branzino is a Mediterranean fish that is sweet, delicious, and perfect for the preparation of this easy-to-prepare* **Salt-Crusted Branzino** *dish.*

**Serves 4 / Serving Size: 1/4 recipe**

# salt-crusted branzino

**2** egg whites

**1/2 cup** kosher salt

**1** whole branzino, cleaned (gutted) with head and tail attached (about 1 1/2 to 2 lb)

1. Whip egg whites to soft peak stage. Stir in salt to make a paste.

2. Rub the paste over the entire fish and roast for 20 minutes until the crust hardens. Let rest for 10 minutes. Crack away the crust and serve only the fish.

## Cook's Tip

*A salt crust on your fish preserves the moisture of the fish. When you crack away the salt crust, only the delicate, moist flavor of the fish remains.*

EXCHANGES/CHOICES: 3 LEAN MEAT
CALORIES 105, CALORIES FROM FAT 20,
TOTAL FAT 2 G, SATURATED FAT 0 G, TRANS FAT 0 G,
CHOLESTEROL 45 MG, SODIUM 75 MG, TOTAL CARBOHYDRATE 0 G,
DIETARY FIBER 0 G, SUGARS 0 G, PROTEIN 21 G

*My go-to ingredients tend to be Italian, but I also find inspiration with Asian flavors, especially for this **Steamed Fish with an Asian Accent** dish.*

**Serves 4 / Serving Size: 1/4 recipe**

# steamed fish with an asian accent

**1/2 cup** orange juice

**2 tsp** light soy sauce

**1 Tbsp** honey

**1/2 cup** sliced scallions (about 1 bunch)

**3 cloves** garlic, sliced into rounds

**1** whole fish (branzino, snapper, salmon), cleaned (gutted) with head and tail attached (about 1 1/2 to 2 lb)

**1/2 lb** snow peas, trimmed

**1 (4 oz) can** sliced water chestnuts, drained and rinsed

**1 (10 oz) can** baby corn, drained and rinsed

1. Mix orange juice, soy sauce, honey, scallions, and garlic in a small bowl.

2. Score the skin on the fish and set fish in steamer basket. Fill the pot with water to the bottom of the steamer basket. Brush 1/2 the sauce over the fish. Cover with lid. Steam for 10 minutes. Add snow peas, water chestnuts, baby corn, and half of the remaining sauce. Cover and steam 3 minutes more. Remove to platter and drizzle with the last of the sauce.

3. Serve with Mushroom Garlic-Scented Rice (recipe on page 153).

## Cook's Tip

*Asian steamer baskets are reasonably priced; however, your stainless veggie steamer will also work well.*

EXCHANGES/CHOICES: 1/2 FRUIT, 2 VEGETABLE, 3 LEAN MEAT
CALORIES 205, CALORIES FROM FAT 20,
TOTAL FAT 2 G, SATURATED FAT 0.4 G, TRANS FAT 0 G,
CHOLESTEROL 45 MG, SODIUM 165 MG, TOTAL CARBOHYDRATE 18 G,
DIETARY FIBER 4 G, SUGARS 12 G, PROTEIN 28 G

# Chapter 9:

# SAUCES AND DRESSINGS

*This **Basic Vinaigrette** can be used as a salad dressing or a marinade. Preparing your own salad dressing is so easy and so much better for you than dressings with preservatives and unpronouncable ingredients.*

**Serves 12 / Serving Size: 1 Tbsp dressing**

# basic vinaigrette

**1/4 cup** vinegar
**2 Tbsp** fresh herbs (chives or basil), chopped (optional)
**1/4 tsp** fine sea salt
**1/4 tsp** freshly ground pepper
**1/2 cup** extra virgin olive oil

1. Place vinegar, herbs, salt, and pepper in bowl. Start whisking and slowly stream in the olive oil. Taste after 1/2 cup has been added. The amount of oil required to balance the vinegar will depend on the vinegar selected.

2. Pour over salads or use as a marinade with chicken, seafood, beef, or any other form of protein you are preparing.

## Cook's Tip

*Slowly whisking in the oil allows for better emulsion.*

EXCHANGES/CHOICES: 2 FAT
CALORIES 80, CALORIES FROM FAT 80,
TOTAL FAT 9 G, SATURATED FAT 1.2 G, TRANS FAT 0 G,
CHOLESTEROL 0 MG, SODIUM 10 MG, TOTAL CARBOHYDRATE 0 G,
DIETARY FIBER 0 G, SUGARS 0 G, PROTEIN 0 G

*This **Basil Pesto Cream** recipe makes a very flavorful and really healthy low-fat dip or spread that your guests will not believe is so good for them! Serve it with grilled or broiled fish or as a dip for crudité.*

**Serves 20 / Serving Size: 1 Tbsp**

# basil pesto cream

**1 cup** fresh baby spinach

**2 cloves** garlic, minced

**1 Tbsp** minced shallot (about 1 large)

**1/4 cup** grated Parmigiano-Reggiano

**1/2 cup** fresh basil

**1 cup** nonfat cottage cheese

**2 tsp** extra virgin olive oil

**2 Tbsp** skim milk (optional)

1. Place spinach, garlic, shallot, Parmigiano-Reggiano, and basil in food processor. Process to a paste.

2. With motor running, add cottage cheese and oil. Process until smooth. Add milk to achieve the desired consistency, if desired.

## Cook's Tip

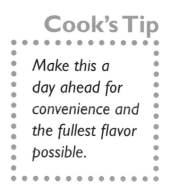

*Make this a day ahead for convenience and the fullest flavor possible.*

EXCHANGES/CHOICES: 1 FREE FOOD
CALORIES 15, CALORIES FROM FAT 5,
TOTAL FAT 0.5 G, SATURATED FAT 0.2 G, TRANS FAT 0 G,
CHOLESTEROL 0 MG, SODIUM 50 MG, TOTAL CARBOHYDRATE 1 G,
DIETARY FIBER 0 G, SUGARS 0 G, PROTEIN 2 G

This **Cilantro & Sunflower Seed Pesto** recipe is absolutely fantastic when you serve it with the Shrimp Quesadilla (page *128*).

## Serves 72 / Serving Size: 1 tsp
# cilantro & sunflower-seed pesto

**2 cups** roasted, unsalted sunflower seeds
**3 cloves** garlic, minced
**1 cup** coarsely chopped fresh cilantro
**4** scallions, chopped
**3 Tbsp** fresh lemon juice
**2 Tbsp** water (additional if necessary)

1. Place seeds, garlic, cilantro, scallions, and lemon juice in food processor fitted with steel blade.  Process to a pureed consistency.

2. Add 2 Tbsp water and process again. The mixture should be a consistency that can be drizzled with a spoon. Extra pesto can be stored in the refrigerator for a few days or frozen.

## Cook's Tip

*Your food processor will make very quick work of this recipe.*

EXCHANGES/CHOICES:  1/2 FAT
CALORIES 20,  CALORIES FROM FAT 20,
TOTAL FAT 2 G,  SATURATED FAT 0.2 G,  TRANS FAT 0 G,
CHOLESTEROL 0 MG,  SODIUM 0 MG,  TOTAL CARBOHYDRATE 1 G,
DIETARY FIBER 0 G,  SUGARS 0 G,  PROTEIN 1 G

*This **Fresh Tomato and Basil Sauce** is a quick no-cook sauce that is great with almost anything, from grilled or broiled fish, to bruschetta and pasta.*

**Serves 16 / Serving Size: 1/4 cup**

# fresh tomato and basil sauce

**12** plum tomatoes, chopped

**2 cloves** garlic, chopped

**1** shallot, minced

**1 Tbsp** extra virgin olive oil

**1/2 tsp** fine sea salt

**1/4 tsp** freshly ground pepper

**1 cup** fresh basil leaves

1. Mix tomatoes, garlic, and shallot. Add olive oil, salt, and pepper. Tear basil leaves and add to tomato mixture.

2. Toss with cooked pasta, serve as a side dish, or use as a bruschetta topping.

## Cook's Tip

*Cook the whole pound of pasta and save half for another meal. Place unsauced pasta in a large plastic bag in the refrigerator for up to 5 days.*

EXCHANGES/CHOICES: 1 FREE FOOD
CALORIES 20, CALORIES FROM FAT 10,
TOTAL FAT 1 G, SATURATED FAT 0.1 G, TRANS FAT 0 G,
CHOLESTEROL 0 MG, SODIUM 75 MG, TOTAL CARBOHYDRATE 2 G,
DIETARY FIBER 1 G, SUGARS 1 G, PROTEIN 1 G

*Pesto* *means paste in Italian. The original Genovese Pesto was made using a mortar and pestle so the texture was not perfectly smooth.*

**Serves 28 / Serving Size: 1 Tbsp**

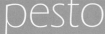
pesto

**4 cloves** garlic

**4 cups** fresh basil leaves (reserve 1 or more sprigs for garnish)

**1/2 cup** freshly grated Parmigiano-Reggiano

**1/2 cup** pignoli (pine nuts)

**1/2 cup** extra virgin olive oil or chicken or vegetable stock

1. Place garlic in food processor and mince. Add basil, Parmigiano-Reggiano, and pignoli and process until smooth. Add olive oil and pulse until well blended.

2. Spoon over Sole Genovese (recipe on page **89**).

## Cook's Tip

*Pesto is so versatile, it's a great idea to make a double batch and freeze half to use with other dishes.*

EXCHANGES/CHOICES: 1 FAT
CALORIES 60, CALORIES FROM FAT 55,
TOTAL FAT 6 G, SATURATED FAT 0.9 G, TRANS FAT 0 G,
CHOLESTEROL 0 MG, SODIUM 10 MG, TOTAL CARBOHYDRATE 1 G,
DIETARY FIBER 0 G, SUGARS 0 G, PROTEIN 1 G

# Chapter 10:

# ROUNDING OUT
# THE MEAL

*This **Asparagus with Orange Vinaigrette** is especially perfect in the spring when asparagus is just coming to the market.*

**Serves 4 / Serving Size: 1/4 recipe**

# asparagus with orange vinaigrette

**2 Tbsp** olive oil
**2 Tbsp** white wine vinegar
**1 tsp** honey
**1/4 cup** chopped shallot (about 1 large)
**1 tsp** dried orange zest
**1 lb** fresh asparagus

1. Heat olive oil in sauté pan. Add white wine vinegar, honey, shallot, and orange zest. Mix well and keep warm for drizzling over asparagus.

2. Place steamer insert in saucepan and add water just until it comes to the bottom of the steamer but not through the holes. Cook until asparagus is fork tender.

3. Lay asparagus on oval platter, and drizzle with vinaigrette. Serve warm or at room temperature.

## Cook's Tip

*Acidulated water, or water mixed with lemon juice, prevents oxidation of sensitive fruits and vegetables like artichokes and apples.*

EXCHANGES/CHOICES: 1 VEGETABLE, 1 1/2 FAT
CALORIES 95, CALORIES FROM FAT 65,
TOTAL FAT 7 G, SATURATED FAT 0.9 G, TRANS FAT 0 G,
CHOLESTEROL 0 MG, SODIUM 10 MG, TOTAL CARBOHYDRATE 7 G,
DIETARY FIBER 2 G, SUGARS 3 G, PROTEIN 2 G

*If you like risotto, why not give this whole-grain version a try. This* **Barlotto with Pesto Ribbons** *is healthier than regular risotto, not to mention delicious.*

**Serves 8 / Serving Size: 1/2 cup**

# barlotto with pesto ribbons

**5 1/4 cups** vegetable stock

**1 1/2 cups** dry white wine

**1 Tbsp** extra virgin olive oil

**1 cup** sweet onion, chopped

**2 cups** barley, checked over for imperfect grains

**1/2 tsp** fine sea salt

**1/2 tsp** freshly ground pepper

**1 large bunch** fresh basil

**1 clove** garlic

**1/4 cup** pignoli (pine nuts)

**1/2 cup, plus 2 Tbsp** freshly grated Parmigiano-Reggiano

**2 Tbsp** finely minced Italian parsley leaves

1. Bring 5 cups vegetable stock and wine to a boil in a 4-quart saucepan. Keep simmering on stove.

2. Using a heavy 4-quart saucepan or chef's pan, add the extra virgin olive oil (thinly film the pan with olive oil), and add onion. Sauté until onion starts to soften. Add barley, salt, and pepper and coat barley grains with olive oil mixture. Add stock mixture 1 cup at a time and stir until each addition of liquid is absorbed.

3. Place basil, garlic, and pignoli in food processor. Add enough vegetable stock to achieve desired consistency—like syrup. Add grated Parmigiano-Reggiano and pulse one or two times. This will create a pesto.

4. When all stock is absorbed and barley is creamy, you can swirl the pesto through like a ribbon. Serve immediately.

EXCHANGES/CHOICES: 3 1/2 STARCH, 1 FAT
CALORIES 320, CALORIES FROM FAT 65,
TOTAL FAT 7 G, SATURATED FAT 1.5 G, TRANS FAT 0 G,
CHOLESTEROL 5 MG, SODIUM 835 MG, TOTAL CARBOHYDRATE 57 G,
DIETARY FIBER 8 G, SUGARS 4 G, PROTEIN 7 G

*Baby artichokes are so handy when you feel like an artichoke in a slightly different style. These **Braised Baby Artichokes** are the perfect side.*

**Serves 6 / Serving Size: 1/6 recipe**

# braised baby artichokes

**16** fresh baby artichokes
Water
**1** lemon, juiced
**1 Tbsp** extra virgin olive oil
**2 cloves** garlic, crushed and peeled
**1 cup** thinly sliced shallots (about 4 medium)
**1 cup** chicken or vegetable stock
**1/4 tsp** fine sea salt
**1/4 tsp** freshly ground black pepper

1. Trim the stem end of the artichokes and remove outer leaves. Cut any prickly points off the artichokes. Place in water with lemon juice to keep from browning. Thinly slice the artichokes vertically (from stem to tip) into 1/4-inch thick slices.

2. Place the extra virgin olive oil in the sauté pan. Add garlic, shallots, and artichokes. Cook 5–10 minutes until vegetables begin to soften.

3. Add 1/2 cup stock, salt, and pepper and cook until tender, about 10 more minutes. Add additional stock to maintain a light sauce layer in the pan.

EXCHANGES/CHOICES: 3 VEGETABLE, 1/2 FAT
CALORIES 85, CALORIES FROM FAT 20,
TOTAL FAT 2.5 G, SATURATED FAT 0.4 G, TRANS FAT 0 G,
CHOLESTEROL 0 MG, SODIUM 315 MG, TOTAL CARBOHYDRATE 15 G,
DIETARY FIBER 8 G, SUGARS 2 G, PROTEIN 3 G

*This* **Couscous & Sun-Dried Tomatoes** *recipe was requested by a friend of mine so that she could have her carbs and protein in one meal.*

---

**Serves 8 / Serving Size: 1/8 recipe**

# couscous & sun-dried tomatoes

**2 cups** chicken or vegetable stock
**1 cup** small dark green lentils
**2 cups** water
**1/2 cup** sun-dried tomatoes (not in oil), cut into bits
**1 Tbsp** Italian seasoning blend
**1 cup** uncooked plain couscous
**1/4 cup** freshly grated Parmigiano-Reggiano

1. Bring 2 cups chicken or vegetable stock to a boil. Add lentils and stir well. Simmer until tender, approximately 20–30 minutes. Be careful not to overcook or they will become mushy. Set aside.

2. Bring 2 cups water to a boil. Add sun-dried tomatoes and Italian seasoning. Simmer 2–3 minutes to soften tomatoes. Bring back to boil. Add 1 cup couscous. Remove pan from heat. Stir and allow couscous to absorb all liquid.

3. Combine couscous and lentils and mix well. Sprinkle with freshly grated Parmigiano-Reggiano.

---

EXCHANGES/CHOICES: 2 STARCH, 1 LEAN MEAT
CALORIES 185, CALORIES FROM FAT 15,
TOTAL FAT 1.5 G, SATURATED FAT 0.5 G, TRANS FAT 0 G,
CHOLESTEROL 0 MG, SODIUM 275 MG, TOTAL CARBOHYDRATE 33 G,
DIETARY FIBER 7 G, SUGARS 3 G, PROTEIN 10 G

*Large grain couscous gives this* Couscous Salad with Roasted Vegetables *more texture but regular couscous also works. Add seafood for a complete meal. Cooked, peeled shrimp would come in handy for this dish.*

**Serves 10 / Serving Size: 1/10 recipe**

# couscous salad
## with roasted vegetables

- **2 cups** couscous
- **4 cups** chicken or vegetable broth
- **8 cloves** garlic, peeled but whole
- **1** small zucchini, cut into 1-inch pieces (about 2 cups)
- **1** small eggplant, chopped into 1-inch pieces (about 2 cups)
- **1** large onion, chopped into 1-inch pieces (about 1 cup)
- **1** green bell pepper, chopped into 1-inch pieces (about 1 cup)
- **1/4 cup, plus 2 Tbsp** extra virgin olive oil
- **3** plum tomatoes, chopped (1 cup)
- **1 Tbsp** fresh oregano, chopped
- **1 Tbsp** fresh basil, chopped
- **1/4 cup** balsamic vinegar
- **1/2 cup** fresh Italian parsley, chopped

1. Preheat oven to 400°.

2. Cook couscous according to package directions, using broth instead of water.

3. Place garlic and vegetables (except tomatoes) in large bowl. Toss with 2 Tbsp olive oil. Place on baking sheet lined with parchment so that they are in one single layer. Roast in oven for 20 minutes or until tender. Cool. Add tomatoes and herbs when vegetables are cooled.

4. Mix couscous and vegetables. Slowly whisk together 1/4 cup oil and vinegar and add to couscous. Mix well. Place on large platter. Garnish with fresh herbs, tomatoes, or sliced oranges.

EXCHANGES/CHOICES: 1 1/2 STARCH, 2 VEGETABLE, 1 1/2 FAT
CALORIES 225, CALORIES FROM FAT 70,
TOTAL FAT 8 G, SATURATED FAT 1.2 G, TRANS FAT 0 G,
CHOLESTEROL 0 MG, SODIUM 400 MG, TOTAL CARBOHYDRATE 34 G,
DIETARY FIBER 3 G, SUGARS 4 G, PROTEIN 5 G

*This **Grilled Vegetables** platter makes a lovely centerpiece for a buffet table. Varying the vegetable types and sizes will add to the appearance of your platter. Serve with just about any dish in this book.*

**Serves 8 / Serving Size: 1/8 recipe**

# grilled vegetables

**1/2 tsp** fine sea salt (divided use)
**1** large eggplant, peeled and sliced into rounds
**2** medium zucchini, peeled and sliced lengthwise
**2** sweet onions, peeled and sliced into very thin rounds
**1** red bell pepper, cored and sliced into rounds
**1** green bell pepper, cored and sliced into rounds
**1** yellow bell pepper, cored and sliced into rounds
**2 Tbsp** extra virgin olive oil
**1/4 tsp** freshly ground black pepper
**2 sprigs** fresh basil (for garnish)

1. Preheat grill or grill pan.

2. Lightly salt eggplant with 1/4 tsp sea salt and let sit for about 10 minutes. Place all vegetables in large bowl and toss with olive oil.

3. Place vegetables on preheated grill and cook to desired doneness. Season with remaining salt and pepper as soon as vegetables are done.

4. Garnish with fresh basil sprigs. Leftover can be used for sandwiches or tossed with pasta.

## Cook's Tip

*Heat kills vitamins and minerals, so the crispier the vegetables the better. Salting the eggplant draws out moisture and forms a moisture barrier to prevent the absorption of too much oil.*

EXCHANGES/CHOICES: 3 VEGETABLE, 1/2 FAT
CALORIES 95, CALORIES FROM FAT 35,
TOTAL FAT 4 G, SATURATED FAT 0.5 G, TRANS FAT 0 G,
CHOLESTEROL 0 MG, SODIUM 155 MG, TOTAL CARBOHYDRATE 16 G,
DIETARY FIBER 4 G, SUGARS 7 G, PROTEIN 2 G

This **Lemon Yogurt Pound Cake** *makes a great presentation when baked in a shaped bundt pan, such as a flower.*

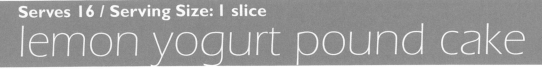

**Serves 16 / Serving Size: 1 slice**

# lemon yogurt pound cake

**1 cup** Splenda

**2 Tbsp** canola oil

**2 Tbsp** lemon zest

**1** lemon, juiced

**1** egg, lightly beaten

**2** egg whites, lightly beaten

**1 cup** plain nonfat yogurt

**2 cups, plus 1 Tbsp** all-purpose flour

**1 Tbsp** baking powder

**1 cup** blueberries

Nonstick cooking spray

**2 tsp** confectioners sugar in a shaker or sifter

1. Preheat oven to 350°.

2. In a large bowl, cream sugar, oil, zest, and lemon juice. Add the egg and egg whites and mix completely. Add yogurt. Combine 2 cups flour and baking powder and add to mixture.

3. Lightly coat blueberries with remaining 1 Tbsp flour. Add blueberries to mixture.

4. Lightly spray cake pan. For cakelette or cupcakes, pour batter in pans to fill 3/4 full. Bake 30 minutes for mini cakes and 50 minutes for large cakes, or until toothpick comes out clean. Sprinkle with confectioners sugar and garnish with blueberries.

EXCHANGES/CHOICES: 1 CARBOHYDRATE, 1/2 FAT
CALORIES 100, CALORIES FROM FAT 20,
TOTAL FAT 2.5 G, SATURATED FAT 0.3 G, TRANS FAT 0 G,
CHOLESTEROL 15 MG, SODIUM 90 MG, TOTAL CARBOHYDRATE 17 G,
DIETARY FIBER 1 G, SUGARS 4 G, PROTEIN 3 G

*Substitute this* **Mashed Celery Root with Garlic** *recipe for garlic mashed potatoes on occasion for a lighter taste treat.*

**Serves 4 / Serving Size: 1/4 recipe**

# mashed celery root with garlic

**2 lb** celery root or celeriac
**2 cloves** garlic
**1/2 tsp** fine sea salt
**1/4 tsp** freshly ground black pepper
**1/2 cup** skim milk
**1/4 cup** chopped flat Italian parsley

1. Cut celery root in quarters or eighths and peel. Place celery root, garlic, salt, and pepper in a 4-quart saucepan and cover with water. Bring to a boil and cook until tender, about 15 minutes.

2. When celery root is done, drain and mash with a large fork or potato masher. Stir in milk and parsley.

## Cook's Tip

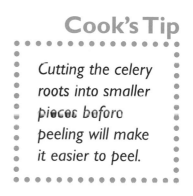

*Cutting the celery roots into smaller pieces before peeling will make it easier to peel.*

**EXCHANGES/CHOICES: 1 STARCH**
**CALORIES 70, CALORIES FROM FAT 0,**
**TOTAL FAT 0 G, SATURATED FAT 0 G, TRANS FAT 0 G,**
**CHOLESTEROL 0 MG, SODIUM 285 MG, TOTAL CARBOHYDRATE 14 G,**
**DIETARY FIBER 3 G, SUGARS 3 G, PROTEIN 3 G**

*These delicious* **Mashed Potatoes** *are even more amazing because you prepare them without cream or butter so they're very healthy.*

**Serves 8 / Serving Size: 1/8 recipe**

# mashed potatoes

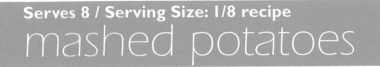

**12** Yukon Gold potatoes, peeled and cut into
1-inch cubes

**1 tsp** fine sea salt

**1/8 tsp** freshly ground pepper

**4 cups** no-salt-added, fat-free chicken, vegetable,
or beef stock

1. Place potatoes, salt, and pepper in heavy saucepan. Add stock and enough water to completely cover potatoes. Boil until potatoes are fork tender, at least 15 minutes.

2. Drain liquid from potatoes into a bowl, and reserve liquid to add back to potatoes.

3. Place potatoes in mixer bowl. Mix until smooth and add some of the stock until potatoes are at the desired consistency.

## Cook's Tip

*Leftover cooking liquid can be used in sauces or soups. These potatoes can be frozen in an ovenproof casserole dish, defrosted, and reheated in a 350° oven until piping hot, approximately 45 minutes.*

**EXCHANGES/CHOICES: 2 1/2 STARCH**
**CALORIES 170, CALORIES FROM FAT 5**
**TOTAL FAT 0.5 G, SATURATED FAT 0.2 G, TRANS FAT 0 G,**
**CHOLESTEROL 0 MG, SODIUM 190 MG, TOTAL CARBOHYDRATE 38 G,**
**DIETARY FIBER 3 G, SUGARS 2 G, PROTEIN 4 G**

*This **Mushroom Garlic-Scented Rice** dish perfectly compliments most of the Asian-style recipes throughout this book.*

**Serves 5 / Serving Size: 1/5 recipe**

# mushroom garlic-scented rice

**1 cup** jasmine rice
**1 clove** garlic, peeled and minced
**2 cups** mushroom broth

1. Place rice, garlic, and mushroom broth in small saucepan. Cover and turn to high. When you see the first sign of steam, turn pan to low and simmer for 25–30 minutes, or as package directs.

## Cook's Tip

*Make this dish more versatile by varying the flavors of stock and by using different herbs.*

EXCHANGES/CHOICES: 2 STARCH
CALORIES 135, CALORIES FROM FAT 0,
TOTAL FAT 0 G, SATURATED FAT 0.1 G, TRANS FAT 0 G,
CHOLESTEROL 0 MG, SODIUM 90 MG, TOTAL CARBOHYDRATE 30 G,
DIETARY FIBER 0 G, SUGARS 0 G, PROTEIN 3 G

*This Orzo Pilaf pasta dish is so incredibly easy because you don't have to boil the pasta separately. It all gets created in one pan.*

**Serves 4 / Serving Size: 1/4 recipe**

# orzo pilaf

**1 Tbsp** extra virgin olive oil

**1 cup** uncooked orzo (rice-shaped pasta)

**2** shallots, minced

**1 clove** garlic, minced

**4 cups** no-salt-added, fat-free chicken or vegetable stock

**1/4 cup** finely minced Italian parsley

**1/4 tsp** fine sea salt

**1/8 tsp** freshly ground black pepper

1. Place olive oil in pan and add orzo. Cook until grains begin to turn golden brown.

2. Add shallot and garlic. Toss well and cook 1–2 minutes.

3. Add 2 cups chicken or vegetable stock and cook on medium until absorbed. Add remaining stock slowly until orzo is cooked, approximately 10 minutes. Add parsley, salt, and pepper to taste.

## Cook's Tip

*Orzo can vary in shape, from short and fat, to long and narrow. The shape variation will also affect the cooking time, so use 10 minutes as a basic guideline.*

EXCHANGES/CHOICES: 2 1/2 STARCH, 1/2 FAT
CALORIES 215, CALORIES FROM FAT 35,
TOTAL FAT 4 G, SATURATED FAT 0.6 G, TRANS FAT 0 G,
CHOLESTEROL 0 MG, SODIUM 280 MG, TOTAL CARBOHYDRATE 37 G,
DIETARY FIBER 2 G, SUGARS 5 G, PROTEIN 6 G

*This delicious **Sautéed Spinach & Garlic** recipe is the easiest side dish you can create at home. It's even easier than a simple salad.*

**Serves 4 / Serving Size: 1/4 recipe**

# sautéed spinach & garlic

**16 oz** baby spinach
**1 clove** garlic, minced
**1 Tbsp** balsamic vinegar or lemon juice (optional)

1. Rinse the spinach in a colander.

2. Place spinach and garlic in a large nonstick skillet. Cook on medium-high heat until spinach is tender, about 5 minutes.

3. Sprinkle with a few drops of balsamic vinegar or lemon juice before serving (optional).

EXCHANGES/CHOICES: 1 VEGETABLE
CALORIES 25, CALORIES FROM FAT 0,
TOTAL FAT 0 G, SATURATED FAT 0.1 G, TRANS FAT 0 G,
CHOLESTEROL 0 MG, SODIUM 90 MG, TOTAL CARBOHYDRATE 4 G,
DIETARY FIBER 3 G, SUGARS 0 G, PROTEIN 3 G

# Index

## Recipes By Alphabetical Order

# Recipes By Subject

# Other Titles from the American Diabetes Association

## Ultimate Diabetes Meal Planner

*by Jaynie Higgins and David Groetzinger*

Fitness and nutrition expert Jaynie Higgins takes the guesswork out of diabetes meal planning and puts everything you need in one amazing collection. With 16 weeks of meal plans and over 300 amazing recipes, this book will guide you toward a healthy, diabetes-friendly lifestyle. You'll find meal plans in four different calorie levels and shopping lists to make grocery shopping a breeze. Take the mystery out of food in just 4 easy steps!

**Order no. 4725-01; Price $21.95**

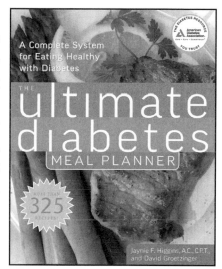

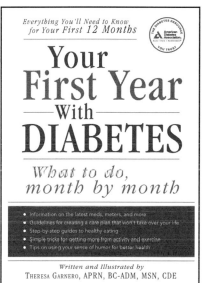

## Your First Year with Diabetes

*by Theresa Garnero, CDE, APRN, BC-ADM, MSN*

Diabetes happens. It can happen to anyone—even you. If diabetes has left you feeling confused or angry, then it's time to turn to Theresa Garnero. Straightforward and easy to read, *Your First Year with Diabetes* will help you manage and deal with your diabetes—day to day, week to week, and month to month. You'll learn about medication, exercise, meal planning, and lifestyle and emotional issues at a pace that suits you.

**Order no. 5024-01; Price $16.95**

## Real-Life Guide to Diabetes

*by Hope S. Warshaw, MMSc, RD, CDE, BC-ADM,
and Joy Pape, RN, BSC, CDE, WOCN, CFCN*

*Real-Life Guide* puts everything you need to know about diabetes into a one-of-a-kind book packed with the information you won't find anywhere else. Learn to prevent long-term complications, understand the ins and outs of health insurance, work physical activity into your daily life, and control your blood glucose, cholesterol, and blood pressure. Bring a realistic approach to your diabetes care plan.

**Order no. 4893-01; Price $19.95**

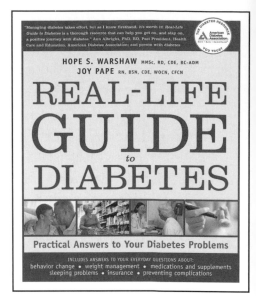

## Diabetes & Heart Healthy Meals for Two

*by the American Diabetes Association
and the American Heart Association*

If you or a loved one has diabetes, you need to eat heart-healthy meals. The simple, flavorful recipes were designed for those looking to improve or maintain their cardiovascular health. Each recipe is for two people, making this book perfect for adults without children in the house or for those who want to keep leftovers to a minimum. With over 170 recipes, there are countless options to keep you heart at its healthiest and your blood glucose under control.

**Order no. 4673-01; Price $18.95**

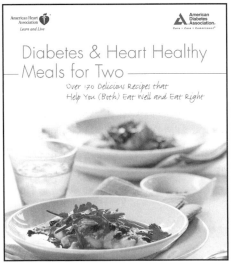

## American Diabetes Association Complete Guide To Diabetes, 4th Edition

*by American Diabetes Association*

Have all the tips and information on diabetes that you need close at hand. The world's largest collection of diabetes self-care tips, techniques, and tricks for solving diabetes-related problems is back in its fourth edition, and it's bigger and better than ever before.

**Order no. 4809-04; New low price $19.95**

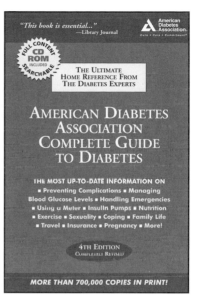

## Guide To Healthy Restaurant Eating, 4th Edition

*by Hope S. Warshaw, MMSc, RD, CDE, BC-ADM*

Eat out without guilt or sacrifice! Newly updated, this bestselling guide features more than 5,000 menu items for over 60 restaurant chains. This is the most comprehensive guide to restaurant nutrition for people with diabetes who like to eat out.

**Order no. 4819-04; Price $17.95**

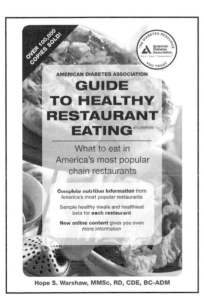

## The Big Book of Diabetic Desserts
### by Jackie Mills, MS, RD
This first-ever collection of guilty pleasures proves that people with diabetes never have to say no to dessert again. Packed with familiar favorites and some delicious new surprises, *The Big Book of Diabetic Desserts* has more than 150 tantalizing treats that will satisfy any sweet tooth.
**Order no. 4664-01; Price $18.95**

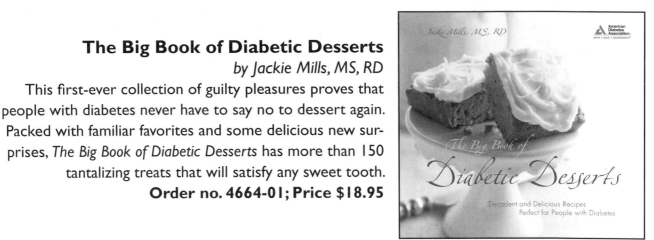

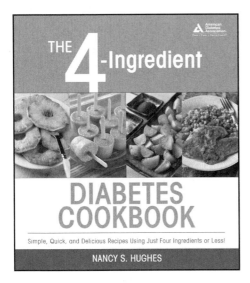

## The 4-Ingredient Diabetes Cookbook
*by Nancy S. Hughes*
Making delicious meals doesn't have to be complicated, time-consuming, or expensive. You can create satisfying dishes using just four ingredients (or even fewer)! Make the most of your time and money. You'll be amazed at how much you can prepare with just a few simple ingredients.
**Order no. 4662-01; Price $16.95**

*To order these and other great American Diabetes Association titles, call 1-800-232-6733 or visit http://store.diabetes.org. American Diabetes Association titles are also available in bookstores nationwide.*